Rare Birds:

The final chapter

A daughter's memoir
Of caregiving in love.

Joan Alexandra Gundersen

First published by Dog Ear Publishing
4010 W. 86th Street, Ste H
Indianapolis, IN 46268
www.dogearpublishing.net

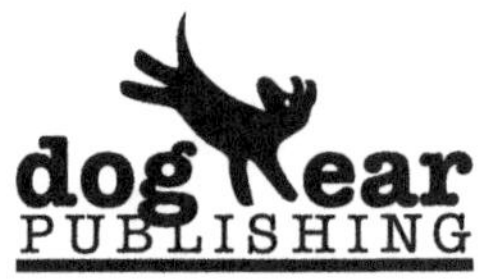

ISBN: 978-1-4575-2695-4

This book is printed on acid-free paper.

Printed in the United States of America

This story is dedicated to my family, Lincoln, Lili, Aksel,
and Christian, that held me during this time,
and to all of Kurt and Maria's helpers.

* Some of the character's names have been changed...just because.

RARE BIRDS: *The Final Chapter*
(A daughter's memoir of her parent's last years)

$\mathscr{T}$he fact that it is 4:00 am and that I have been called awake from REM sleep by my frail and helpless mother – is the way it is, under the circumstances. Kurt, my dad, is still living at home at 82 with Alzheimer's dementia for 6 years. I'd guess he is mid-stage in the progression of the disease. He lives independently (with an army battalion of help) in his 2-bedroom bungalow in La Crosse, Wisconsin with my mother – his wife Maria. Theirs is a deeply entwined marriage of 43 years – my own age. I was born right after they exchanged vows. Their union always central and strong was a second for them both and one of rare true love and devotion. My sister and I just rode along on the bus, subject to our parents. We learned ways to cope as children.

Tonight, when my mother called me – was the beginning of a new phase of problems in my father's failing condition. She heard him struggling on the floor, unable to stand up. Usually the home aides (thank God for them) find him lying there on his back with a pillow under his head, wrapped with whatever he can find – a carpet, a towel, a pad – whatever he can readily grab will suffice as a blanket. The difficulty in finding him is not the initial surprise (scare?) but it is in the helping him to get up, to stand up again.

I didn't realize the difficulty until tonight when I rushed down from deep slumber on a rainy fall night, to find him seated on the bathroom floor. He tried to use the sink and toilet to help him stand; sometimes, even amusing himself by playing with the toilet water, fully dressed but stuck, struggling to get up from the floor. My mother yelling, "Oh, I didn't mean it to be you Joanie! Call April, the nursing assistant or call John the neighbor, or a police officer or two!" It sounds like planning for the tea parties my mother loved to have. (This was the guest list.)

My Mother is a World War II survivor, a British citizen and very fond of tea anytime, anywhere, with anyone, for all situations. Tonight she can't get him to stand on his feet, to support himself. You see the simplest task becomes complicated. My dad takes a tumble. "There are two of them", he says. Who or what are "them" I wonder. He is so sure they are a part of his world. "Let's get up" I tell him, "Give me your hand." He loves to grip tightly. It shows us his strength and power, his past dominance or attempted dominance - a game he played with us as children. He had to deal with me and I did not accept his orders, always. Well, let's not go to the past. For now there is the task at hand.

I turn on classical music. It soothes him and speaks to him more then any other voice. Maybe it will tell him how to stand. Maybe it will help him to unscramble. Nevertheless, it is beautiful and soothing to me at 4am with a head cold. I am there. April has resorted to a Guernsey to hoist him up. "Let him rest on the sofa if he likes", mom yells. He has a way of sleeping sitting up and listening to classical radio music. Tonight we decide to put him back to bed fully clothed with shoes to help him stand should he need to again.

"Want, listen to the music." He says as he makes his way back to bed. "It's sleep time." I say. He has had his days and nights mixed up for days. "Sundowners" it's called. He is active at night and prefers to be nocturnal it seems. This moving on the floor in crab or snake fashion is a new one. At least he's not wandering for miles from home, across town – a phase he went through a year ago. The fear of not knowing where he was and possibilities of his endangerment was terrible. He has evolved into the latter stages of Alzheimer's dementia since then.

"Go to hell." He tells me as April tucks him in. The anger swells and falls. "It's OK" April responds. We find to agree with him comforts him. "Oh daddy, what has become of you?" He is forever lost to another time. Really, there is no retrieving him now. I must be grateful to have what is left of him, his anger and strength. I ask how long can we all go on like this? What if I had a job to face the next morning? I wouldn't be able to handle the p.m. calls. I will awake to a house of 6 children, my 3 and their overnight guests. That will be more manageable than a full-blown career, other then the fact that I will bite of their heads with my tiredness. I don't have a real job, but I can be there for them and it is what matters to me. I accept them as my day job but not my night job too! Tomorrow I will check for respite care for her by signing my father up for Adult day care just a few mornings per week.

2

"*D*arling, come and sit closer to me and listen to Wagner. It's *The Flight of the Valkaries.*" Maria, now 76, scoots her wheelchair over by Kurt. She has not yet given into the electric jazzy tilt-a-chair that empowers her but also weakens the little muscle she has left. She has been ravaged by Rheumatoid Arthritis, which she has had for half of her being. I believe it resulted from the stress of surviving her WW2 escape from Poland, through the iron curtain. He does what he loves best, conducting Wagner's music from the living-room sofa. It is the same sofa his parents had in their Philadelphia home after emigrating from Germany in 1922, soon after Kurt was born. He had been too big a baby, demanded too much from his mother Minna, or "Mutti" (mother in German) as he called her, and many others. They left Germany for a better life in America. Kurt was raised as a child amongst adults by his grandparents, Sophia and Wilhelm Klie. This may have been the seed of his chronic anger, angst that he always exhibited and rarely hid. He never tried to make a good impression on a new acquaintance. He was verbal, intelligent and quick to anger. What you saw was what made up Kurt, throughout. I think his friends appreciated the honesty of his being.

I came daily once or twice, (or when called in an emergency) to check on their well-being since their recent move from the suburbs of Washington D.C. to God's Country, La Crosse, Wisconsin, a town in the midst of bluffs and a river. This was my new home where I was raising our three children with my physician husband, Lincoln. Kurt's favorite aspect of Midwestern living was the 'fresh air,' he commented on this regularly, "What good air it is today."

"Mom, should I turn the hot water on for tea? Do you want green or black today? How was your doctor's appointment?"

Kurt is still on the sofa, passionately conducting Wagner or now his beloved Puccini, and his opera "Nessun Dorma" in Turondot. His eyes tear up during the final stanza, "I shall win!" he wales in Italian. He acquired a taste for opera, growing up in Germany it was an entertainment offered to the community Kassel, in the throes of war.

"Maria, can't you tell her to shut up?"

I'm in the middle of something! 'What's all this hocus pocus?'

"Damn it. What's the matter with you people." His gruff voice resounded enhanced with heavy German annunciation[1]

I roll my eyes but know after years of being Kurt's daughter; his 'number one' he would call me, that it is not worth arguing with him. A temper-tantrum may ensue. Maria and I go to the front room, a kind of sunroom in the front of the small prairie-style bungalow that is now their Wisconsin home: 330 S. 21st street, on a tree lined street with a wide sidewalk. I found the house for them and they came from the D.C. area to their new home sight unseen. They trusted my word as their 'number one' daughter. This would be the home where they would spend their golden years. The most desirable feature was that the alley and a white picket fence that is all that really divided my home from theirs. There were many hot meals and treats that were shuttled back and forth between our big yellow wooden Victorian house and theirs. This was idyllic really, until Kurt's Alzheimer's progressed to mid-stages and he decided to prune our bushes, bush shredding instead of shearing, with his bare hands. This special service included reaching beyond our yard to the neighbors. The scope of this activity included flower picking, fence supervision and control, and tree maintenance. Many times he would wander off into the alley and return with beautiful bouquets of wild flowers, alley shrubs and also neighbor's garden flowers for his beloved Maria. My mother was very touched by this sweet act of devotion until an enraged neighbor's voice would call one of us to complain. Some would scream so

---

[1] As much as he tried to lose this after the war in his quest for Americanization, he never really did.

loudly, I had to hold the phone 5 inches from my ear, " You must control your father. He was in my yard again! He needs 24 hour care. My petunias have been destroyed." Or another day, "Your father is a menace. Next time he comes over to manage the fence builders work in our yard we are calling the police!" Somehow these vindictive voices added insult to the injury, the wound that was already there in dealing with my father's demise. In my mind, I thought, "Fence building supervisor." What an ideal job for a retired engineer.

Looking back, I think his passion for fence control not only was a result of his boredom but due to the war years' effect on him with its mandates. Born in 1920, in Kassel, Germany, he clearly recalled WWI and Hitler's control over his native country. He explained once to me that the impending Hitler regime with all of its zealousness somehow left him feeling threatened. He sensed that the absolute power this leader was expecting was somehow askew. Kurt was a stellar student, and when he was around the age of 15, the Nazi youth group invited him to join. The head master told Kurt, '"If you go to America, good German blood will be lost." Being leery of the movement, he knew it was time to join his parents in America. Oscar Happe, his father, had established himself as a diesel engineer for Baldwin Locomotive in Philadelphia; Millie, his wife, worked as a hairdresser in her own small beauty parlor. They lived in a large and dark pillared row house on Springfield road, not too far from Drexel University where Kurt applied his gift for math to become an engineering graduate. This included special training at MIT in radar. He applied this in China (1943) in a military intelligence mission; he rose to the rank of lieutenant colonel. In Boston, during his studies, he resided with an Episcopal minister who must have converted him to Episcopalianism, that his been our religion ever since.

3

I had the inclination to take Kurt to church yesterday. When the inclination hits, I become certain it is the right thing to do and nothing will stop me. He hasn't been in months, I reasoned. It is always a challenge to get him up and ready by the first hymn so we usually make the second, or the sermon at least. Ours is the back pew, where we have more privacy to express our religion, and commune with one another. The sermon ends about reality and holiday expectations/ Advent etc. We are on to the Apostles' Creed and Kurt bellows the "Amens" loudly and sings along to the hymns. He's rather put together today in his gray polar fleece and driving "cappy" as he calls it, all, but the scrubby hair and unshaven face- the male R.N. probably did the best he could without being insulted and accused, because of Kurt's bad mood.

He seems to be content singing and sitting with the congregation as they do humming along in the next hymn, until I hear a loud trickle, like a fountain or summer hose spray. I freeze in shock, thinking I thought he went to the bathroom this morning and mom says he's under control! The only one bothered by it is the lady in the pew ahead of us who slides over causally. I changed many diapers in the exact pew many times, why was it so different? I calmly go to the coffee cart to grab a wad of napkins. He is smiling contentedly when I return, Quickly I wipe up the puddle yet don't disturb the stain on his wet pants. Luckily this happened during the world prayers since I know the minister will offer to bring communion to him today for his walking is slow and unsteady. As I cover up evidence of the accident and plan our exit, Father and the

7

acolytes approach us looking calmly. Did they see the watery dark stain on his pants? I do smell an odor. Just cool and calmly, after receiving bread, we are free. Who knows what could happen next. I question if we will go to church ever again.

Maria would wait patiently at home for the after church delicacies that we would bring to her for her late breakfast. Due to her severe Rheumatism, she seemed to prefer to lie in bed until at least 10 a.m. to give time for the strong pain pills to kick in. The Oxycontin and Loretabs were her anecdote to this extreme suffering – taking up to 10 a day. Although she refused to be bedridden, she was frozen in her bed until an aide would come to her assistance to help her rise, towel bathe, and then be hoisted or hoyer lift into her chair. By the time I came in mid-morning, she was usually completely put together for the day's routines and visitors. One of her helpers (there were up to 50 total in these last years as so many came and went due to burn out or agency shifts) Rebecca, a Mary Kay lady on the side, would leave her stamp on Maria by always dressing her in pink. "I just love pink, it is the color for a princess, which of course we all are," she would banter.

Not only was Rebecca a Mary Kay lady but also an aspiring novelist on the side. When I finally was invited to read one of her novels, I noted their harlequin romance quality – very raw and steamy. I thought of my proper mother, very Victorian in her being, probably enjoying this exciting slant on her new Wisconsin life. Maria was born in Victorian England in 1923. The daughter of a "Baltic" Estonian/Swede Navy man – a member of the Royal Navy – Karl Von Dehn ended up being captain of the Royal Yacht Standart to the Tsar Nicholas and his son Alexander. Maria's beloved mother Lili Dehn, wrote a memoir "The Real Tsarista" from her perspective of the Tsar's wife, the illusive Alexandra, bringing a greater intimacy to her person. Maria had high standards to live by in her degree of civility but she bowed gracefully to her more down to earth Wisconsin world of the 1990's, where 'anything goes.' She became kind of a moral pillar of steel for all of those around her to lean on. She had an ear for all of our problems and gave each of us her profound wisdom based on what was proper from her Victorian days and also her earthy wisdom gained from having survived an escape through the iron curtain of Poland, losing her possessions time and again, (see page 122) only to reinvent herself in her new surroundings. Whether it was the finishing school she attended in France or the exotic world of post-war Venezuela where her family finally fled to after the German invasion of Poland.

I always thought it was ironic that she married my father, a German native, after her war flight away from the Germans. But it was love at first sight at her family get-together in Caracas. Kurt's first wife, the Baroness Von Guenderrode, had expressed her desire to leave him out of her own dissatisfactions. He had swept her away once, from her small town near Frankfurt when he drove through as an American Officer on a reconnaissance mission to bandage some of the damages of war bombed Germany. Caroline or Roli as we called the baroness, was one of the first American-German was brides after their encounter. With her inability to bear a child and her desire to live in Colorado, Kurt was given a green light to pursue her cousin Maria, who was also married for two years to her Polish sweetheart Karl. She tried to ignore Kurt's advances but her own dissatisfaction with her marriage and spoiled husband's demands also led her to see his innuendos as a new opportunity. The fact that Kurt was now an American German who had left his German home for a successful engineering job in the U.S. must have also appealed to her. This was a stable man, someone with whom she could finally have a family. Although it took months of Kurt's aggressive wooing to finally win her over, Maria agreed finally to an international divorce against her Catholic ex-husband's wishes. She was forced to leave everything behind – her family (mother, brother, sister and friends) so she could clear a path for Kurt and herself in America. She had expressed the meaningless quality of material things over and over to us as a lesson that she had taken with her, having learned to leave all possessions, homes, cars, and even loved ones behind in pursuit of safety, personal freedom and a promise of a better life ahead. As a result of their escapade I came to be; She carried me in the dusty streets of Mexico until her papers were cleared for her immigration to Washington D.C. where Kurt waited for her and I was born a bit early…but a blessed child nevertheless.

Blessed to have such marvelous and loving parents. My upbringing took me to Rome where we resided for five years and then to D.C., where my parents in the suburbs of Bethesda, Maryland raised me and my sister, Marina.

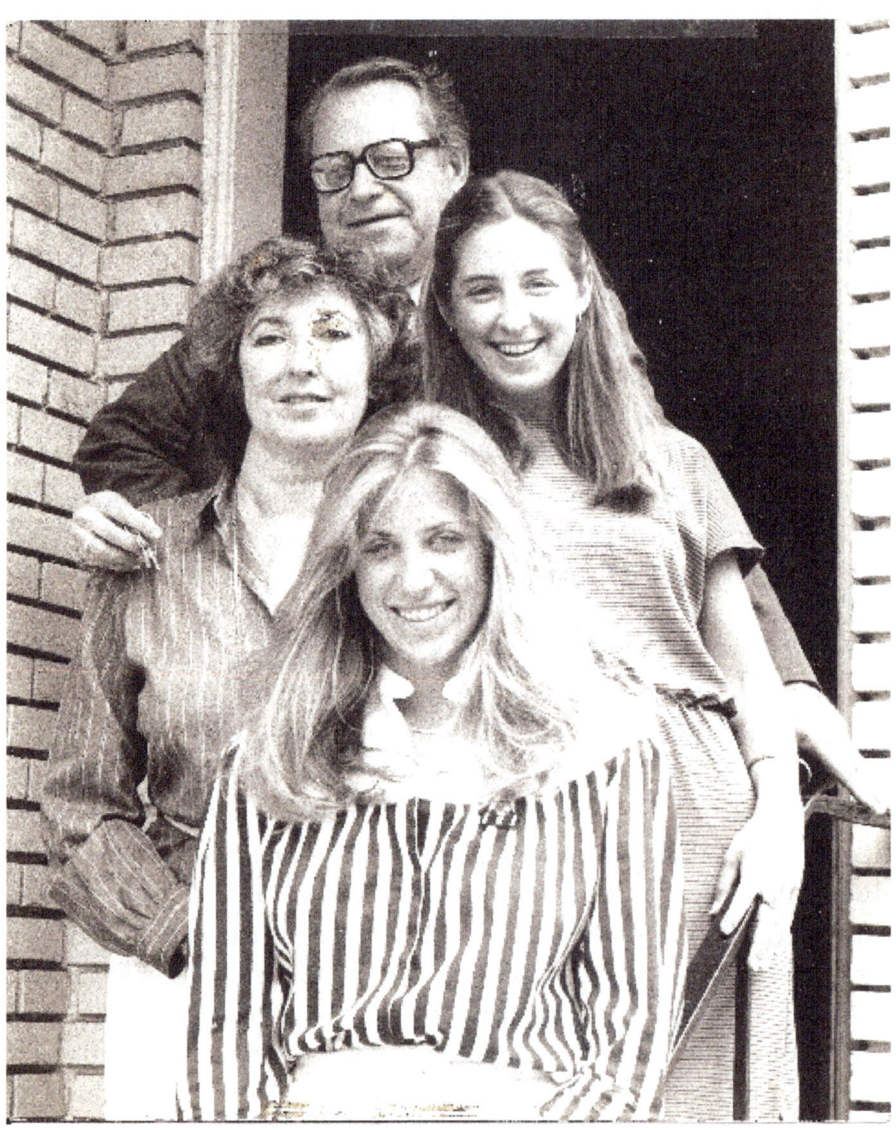

Our family in the 80's: Kurt, Maria, Marina, and Joanie

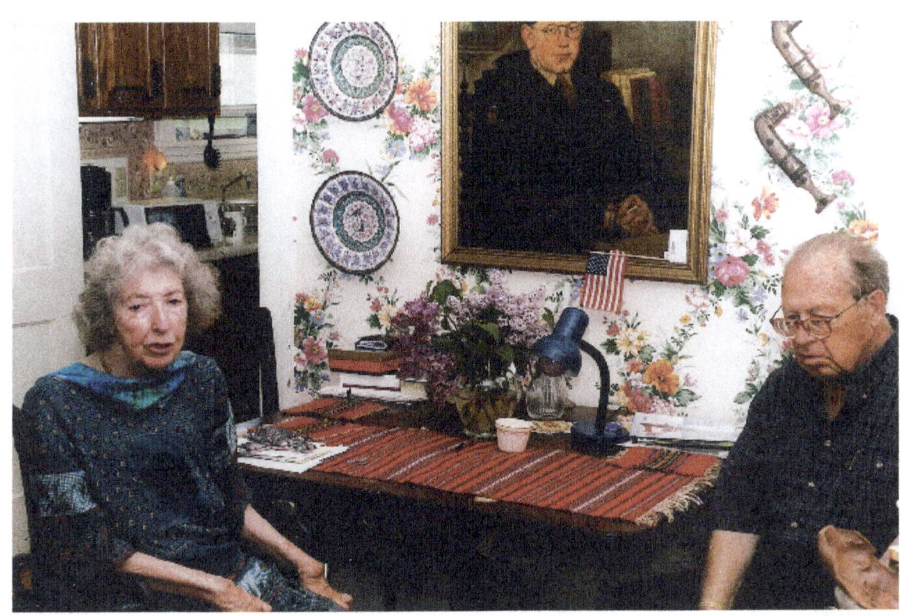

Kurt and Maria in their Wisconsin home

4

*M*y parents and their old world European ways were always of interest to my all-American friends. For one thing their Northern European cooking included dishes such as Borscht, green sauce from Germany, cabbage rolls and some German sausage dishes.[2]

The scents from the kitchen were always overpowering for any of my suburban American friends who preferred canned tomato soup, grilled cheese and coke for lunch. Maria kept up this style of cooking after Kurt was gone, and it was always just as good, made with the help of the staff of three to four home health-aids who she trained to prepare these dishes. In the past she was the sous -chef in her own kitchen and Kurt was the main cook. She would suggest spices and ingredients in their order while he did the food prep. Although he was a natural cook, (his stout shape verified this) he was very dependent on her input for many old world recipes.

On one occasion, one of my favorite neighbor boys dropped by and my father was in the kitchen making a chicken stock. Jim tells the story of how he came across a burly, gruff German man, doggedly pulling apart a chicken. It must have terrified him because Jim did not call back for any more dates with me, to my chagrin.

The green sauce recipe, which I have included, is in the recipe section in the back. It was the most sacred and challenging recipe of their unified cooking. This German recipe required the use of the

---

[2] See recipes in appendix.

freshest spring herbs available and when finished, it was a kind of homemade mayonnaise-herb sauce to be served over basic potatoes and meat. Beer was a must with this spring tonic recipe. In their case, it always included a visit from the grune sauce expert, Aunty Roli, Baroness Von Guenderrode. They always told us that the reason they split was because Roli did not want children and was determined to reside in Aspen, Colorado, to live the life of an avid skier. Their cats were their surrogate children. I guess the reason for her continued visits in Kurt's new life with my mother was related to the fact that Roli was Maria's second cousin; she also had a family tie to Maria. We were what she had left of family.

Roli came bi-yearly and usually traveled with a cat. Mitzi-lion and her low purr (growl) inhabited the basement room. Roli poked holes in her travel bag so that Mitzi-lion could survive the trans-Atlantic trip. I will forever recall her heavy German accent, and brassy orange hair, as she called out necessary tips and ingredients for the spring grune sauce recipe. Her brash cackle when my father overlooked something, "That is why I left him. He was too controlling! How do you all deal with this?"

Maria would simply let the insults pass as she sat in her regal way, but her look and solemn face would let one know that she was clearly not overjoyed by the family guest. Over the years, Roli's hair grew brighter and brighter red as her personality became more outlandish. One of the more embarrassing incidents that I can't forget due to my young disapproval was the fact that my European parents – more down to earth and practical than my American friends – refused to have curtains on their windows, or if they did, they were sheer and rarely shut in order to let the sunlight in. They would carelessly change into their nightclothes (actually they dressed scantily creating a peepshow of sorts for bored neighborhood kids.)

Kurt was always focused on the "Jewish solution" and the Israeli Palestine conflict in the 70's and 80's. He posed this question to their dinner table guests frequently and rambled on often heatedly about this world conundrum. He often mentioned that this hot spot and conflict would resonate into WW3, and cause major destruction and upheaval. So far, it has not been the cauldron he claimed, but that is not to say it couldn't have potential. His parents Oscar and Minna Happe left Germany to make a better life in America but this decision had been fueled by Hitler's totalitarian regime and their personal distrust of it. This explained Kurt's chronic 'doom and gloom' attitude about the world's potential end.

It was difficult to be a German-American residing in Washington D.C. in the post-war years, especially if one had a heavy German accent. He felt this subtle discrimination and often had to undergo government confidential security checks for his work in order to navigate freely in the US and abroad. As engineer marketing satellite equipment to the mid-east, he must have appeared as a suspicious character quite often. I think he envied Henry Kissinger's success in the US government and often wished for his own political savvy would take him further. Due to these insecurities as an American-German, always seen as a foreigner in his chosen land, he refused to teach my sister and I German in the hope that we would be true, blue Americans. I regretted this decision. I studied German in college and even beyond in my later years. Yet, my father's wish has prevailed, and my German is terrible! He would spend hours correcting my poor grammar as I practiced with him whenever possible.

"Maria, this is terrible. She is pulling my leg."

In reality it was just my poor attempt at speaking my father's language.

5

Kurt's Alzheimer's

*M*aria believes it all began in his 70's, when she noted that he showed very little interest in the selling of their family home in order for them to join my family in Wisconsin. Normally, very money conscious, Kurt cared little about the monetary transaction and house sale. Here is a photo of Kurt satisfied with the recent Bethesda house sale.

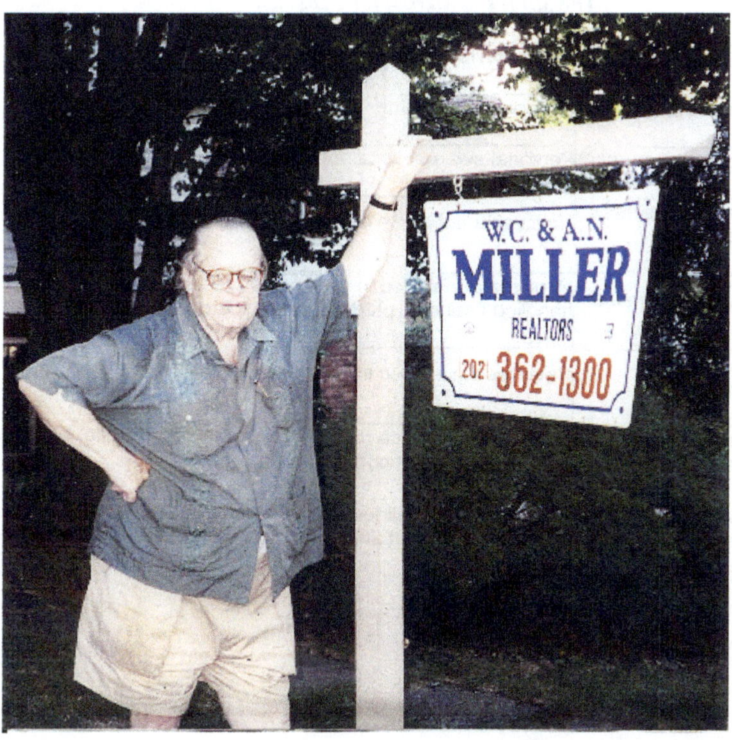

After a few gentle months in Wisconsin his seven-year demise began. I only noted his strange lack of engagement in our phone conversations. "Yes dear, yes dear", in a proper European accent- in an almost drugged sense, where it seemed what I was saying was not being registered.

Although his demise from this point took a total of about seven-years from when he was officially diagnosed with Alzheimer's dementia, my mother and I were proud to say that we, with the band of community helpers, who would come and go in shifts from their two bedroom prairie style bungalow, were able to keep Kurt in a home and familiar setting for this whole 6-7 year period. He progressed through most of the stages of Alzheimer's according to the FAST scale[3], without having to live in a care center until the <u>very last 3 months of his life</u>, but simply with the home care that my mother and I, and eventually a caseworker, were able to manage. We had many glorious moments with my colorful father; yet also some that were inglorious, as previously described.

The Stages of Alzheimer's Disease

FAST Scale Stage	Characteristics
1... normal adult	No functional decline.
2... normal older adult	Personal awareness of some functional decline.
3... early Alzheimer's disease	Noticeable deficits in demanding job situations.
4... mild Alzheimer's	Requires assistance in complicated tasks such as handling finances, planning parties, etc.
5... moderate Alzheimer's	Requires assistance in choosing proper attire.
6... moderately severe Alzheimer's	Requires assistance dressing, bathing, and toileting. Experiences urinary and fecal incontinence.
7... severe Alzheimer's	Speech ability declines to about a half-dozen intelligible words. Progressive loss of abilities to walk, sit up, smile. and hold head up

The Fast Scale

In addition to his yard art, Kurt created a magical world of found material and ice-sculptures in their picket-fenced backyard, during the frozen winter months by turning on the hose in the frosty air. A spiral pattern was created in the icy grass. (See photos of Kurt's ice art on page 19).

Paddhie Kurt's aide, would stay with my father through his late night antics.

"Your father was up all night. We played the faucet game; he would turn it on and then I would turn it off. After that we danced a bit to the radio tunes," Paddhie would say.

Luckily Maria removed her hearing aids at night and did not hear the party that these two had.

"Then he conducted some music for me while I played the pots and pans." Paddhie had a melancholy, introverted streak, which eventually turned out to be unidentified schizophrenia, unknown to us.

One day we come home to one of Paddhie's solemn states. All of the pictures around our home had been flipped about to face the back wall, and all our alcohol stock emptied down the drain. (She found alcohol to be an un-pure thing, so she made it vanish.) She was dressed very daintily in a bright orange outfit and hat. She had packed her things. Her condition clarified- she had not been taking her medications and she was becoming too remote and strange.

Her ride came to return her to her residence in Madison and to a treatment center. We were distraught. Where would we find a night helper to care for Kurt in this entertaining way again?

Soon after she departed, Kurt's life did end; and the missing portrait of Kurt in his American Army uniform, which hung in a central spot in their home that was amiss, was symbolic of the nearing future event. That is why I described Paddhie as angelic, and even prophetic.

Although we still had Kurt's' beloved helper April on staff (a young mother of 3), we had to come up with another night one to help with the evening shift and Kurt's sundowners.

I often would find April and Kurt sitting on the sofa, listening to Wagner. Kurt would spend hours conducting it. Another favorite was the Classical music of Rachmaninoff and Chopin, which never failed to appease him. As we were growing up, we were subjected to hours of Opera.

I think this phase is his music taste was an improvement. April would usually hold his hand. He would say, "You love me don't you. You are my sweetheart."

Maria would notice them both sitting so smugly together and look on disapprovingly with a bewildered glance. She chose to tolerate this as she did many things. She was extremely tolerant throughout her life.

April became a main stay in the house as Maria relied on her physically and Kurt- mentally. Her famous statement, which came after much experience as a CNA was: "You know, Kurt has the freedom to fall." This was very thought provoking. Maybe it was a good way out of the horrific cycle that lay ahead.

I previously shared about his tendency of tree and bush shredding; my hard working medical husband looked very dismayed when he came home one day to find a mangled mulberry tree in our backyard. My mother also seemed very discouraged one afternoon when she pointed out the distorted poinsettias and other potted garden plants that she had grown. I do recall he had this tendency to over-trim things at our Maryland home.

Often my mother would call over in a panic to tell me that Kurt had disappeared. One of the behaviors of an Alzheimer's individual is their tendency to wander. One second he would be in eye's view in the yard and then another gone. With his walking stick and battered "Door County touristy cappy" on, as he would call it, walking stick in hand, and dog on a leash in the other, he would be off on these many neighborhood adventures. A few times he would make himself at home at another residence and have to be brought home by the police. My biggest fear was that he would wander into the Mississippi River- and that would be his ending. The poor old Westie that Kurt aimlessly walked, was truly a devoted creature. He never left Kurt's side on these meanderings, even when they walked to far neighborhoods, miles astray. Only after this year phase of "traveling", as Kurt would describe it- did the Alzheimer Association come up with a cap or band with a microchip or tag telling the friends Kurt found on the way how to "return" him, and Winnie the Westie to his proper place. After one adventure, I found Kurt back home after being saved by the

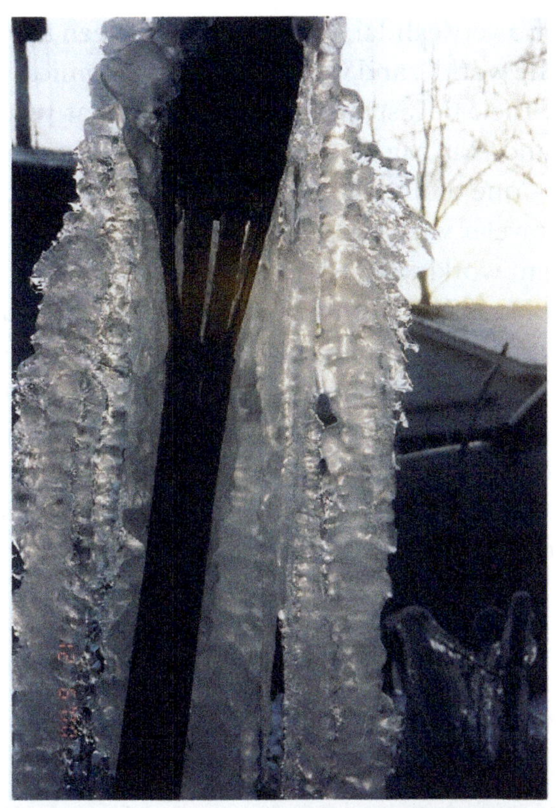

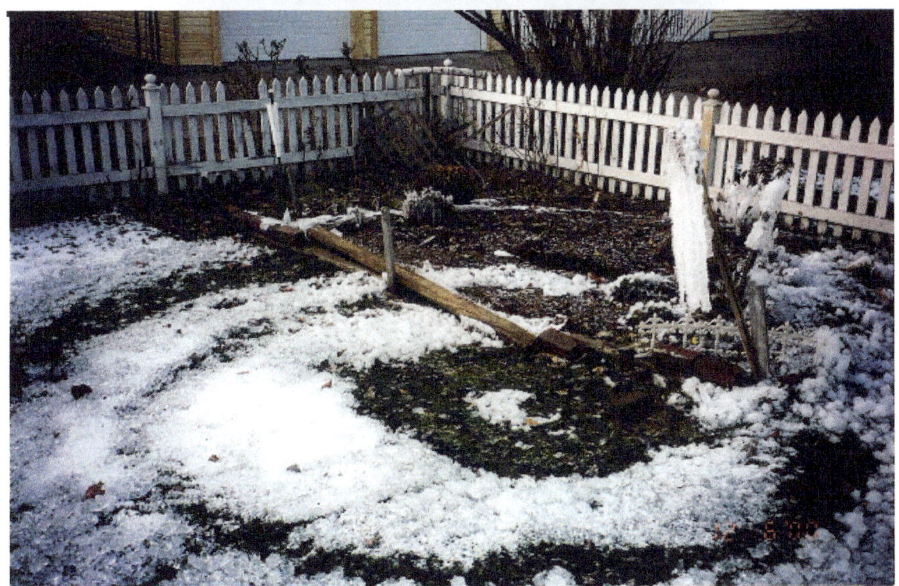

Yard ice art creations by Kurt

police again, in a very exhilarated state; "I have been traveling…I have been all over the world", and with his angry but comical edge, "China, India, Burma, the Mideast" – all these places that you people have never been", and "Ma Ma Fu Fu, horse, horse, tiger, tiger", from his China period – one of his favorites. There was a grain of truth in this, for he was a traveler with his job in marketing satellite communications equipment working all over the world.

Towards the end of his life, Kurt would move around their bed and say, "What does she do for me?" He would then proceed to take apart Maria's wheelchair and borrow her clothes. I would often find Kurt looking exasperated at the edge of the bed wearing her floral design cremeline shirt which clearly did not fit and her wheelchair's parts all over the floor. Some days he would tug on her sore leg like a small boy trying to roust his mom. Maria had the patience of a saint, as she would helplessly await for a helper to save her.

6

here were a slew of helpers that were always at my parent's side. I, and my mother in her invalid state were the first to admit that we could not manage Kurt alone. We knew there was "lockdown" facilitates available but somehow the overriding goal was to maintain his integrities and some priviledges of freedom, and moving there would have been somewhat debilitating; it surely would have disoriented him and possibly diminished his free movement, which somehow seemed important. We did have a trial at a lockdown place- a unit or wing at the local care centers. Kurt would visit there one to two times a week, on a drop-in basis, to give Maria a bit of a respite. Alzheimer's has been called the 48-hour job, with the intensity of a supervisor required! Yet, after a few time of Kurt's visits, the staff complained of his being belligerent and needing to be medicated on his visits. I did not want to see him in an overly calm and zombie-like state, and I was not keen on extra drugs and their affects regulating him. I knew he was sensitive, as the time he was on *Haladol due* to a Congestive Heart Failure incident, which made him completely crazy. The hospital made it clear to me that this was not the route to go on with Kurt. It clearly agitated and confused him. Soon he was discharged from the day care, due to our resistance to the drugs. The strangest recollection I have of this time is of the other residents (with dementia) holding baby dolls and stuffed-animals always announcing my arrival like this- "Kurt your son is here to pick you up." Maybe my father has always wished for a son, and they all knew.

I had a family and three children in the middle-range years that required much attention. My husband, who always seemed to be a family man, could only participate so much in this world due to his demanding medical job and he soon burned out. One of our favorite helpers was named "Paddhie", (as mentioned previously) an unusual configuration for Patty; she came to us like an angel out of the mist. As always, we simply put an ad in the local paper and the responses would come to our call. Often it was just 1 or 2 individuals that had responded to our caregiver ad, in exchange for room and board. Paddhie was a dear elderly woman, with a lot of zest and flippant way about her that somehow endeared my father to her. She had a rare patience of a mystical sort. After all, the Alzheimer individual's day was a 48-hour one and most of the caregivers were often suffering from extreme fatigue. Paddhie seemed to be the most resilient. She would describe her nights with Kurt, who was up for many hours of them, while the rest of us were asleep: "Lots of water play, tapping, and music making."

Maria always had a few things by her bed on the night-table: Ricola cough drops, a glass of water, a back-scratcher, half a orange for dry mouth, all to aide her in times of wanting or being stranded between helpers. (That must have been many hours, where aides were late due to car or personal problems, or weather issues.)

Even Dan, the so-called "base," may not have been available on the scene due to meetings with his social worker or parole officer, (he had been delinquent with his child-support payments,) or occasional day jobs at the canoe building factory, for instance. His only required duty was the night block in exchange for free rent.

One day, I even had to break into their home due to Dan having been in jail (apprehended for delinquent child support payments,) 5 hours north of town. Maria was found alone in bed, patient and peaceful as always, waiting for a very late a.m. helper who was to get her out of bed, dress her, and feed her.

Transitioning Maria was a huge ordeal and a Hoyer lift was required. Helpers spent hours of training to man this iron workhorse of a machine. It required precise maneuvers or Maria would seethe in pain. I often would find her in a cocoon mode, hanging in the sling, waiting for assistance of any kind.

Dan was a miracle as he treasured Maria and worked only in exchange for room and board. It was as if we wished him. He came on board after Kurt's passing and charmed us all. He was Maria's very own lifeline. He allowed for her to live at home and not in a care-center. We simply put an ad in the local newspaper, and he was one of the few that personally responded.

In order to revive Baba, the Russian name for grandmother that she chose for herself, I would take Kurt on weekly outings when he was still more mobile. This would give her a necessary reprieve. Once he visited a Shakespeare outdoor theater for a summer production of *As You Like It*. Kurt insisted on wearing the program booklet wide open as a hat. I think the flying nun wore her habit like this. An even greater embarrassment was his sudden need to urinate under a tree during intermission on our way to the restroom. Many people, especially women, gave us disappointing looks, and I don't blame them. I was flabbergasted, as he was often unmanageable, like this time.

I knew Maria was worn thin trying to cope with her own condition and then to manage Kurt's care, but she insisted on caring for him. It surely was a labor of love and a result of her iron will and disciplined character. One must take care of one another, even on sinking ships, and this is what 330 S. 21st felt like sometimes, a sinking ship with the Captain Kurt, going down fighting. I even had a dream of this nature once, which remains vivid in my mind. Kurt is swirling down in a river of water as if in a drain, yet his fist remains thrust in the air despite his disappearance swirling into the funnel of water. This reminded me of a "Figa" a Brazilian luck charm that he once gifted me with from his foreign travel.

7

The Helpers:

There was a battalion of helpers involved in my parents care. I was most impressed with their loyalty and devotion to the cause, as I am sure that the pay was minimal and the burnout rate-high. Some came from local agencies as CNA'S or CNA assistants, and others just came as if by magic and would answer our beckon calls, through word of mouth or otherwise: April, Laura, Barb, Berta and Juan, Vladamina, Rebecca, Marilyn, Jane, Ron (who was like a personal valet), Paddhie, and Dan.

Dan

He resembled Maria's son-in-law, almost as if he was a brother-not so much in character, but appearance. His big warm, brown eyes asked us to trust him. He exuded caring and kindness.

Maria and Dan instantly took to one another. All seemed clear for Maria to be able to return home (despite the social worker's disapproval) after Kurt's death and her 6 months recuperation at a care center. Even I was becoming skeptical of her ability to manage alone.

Dan came on the scene and it seemed everything would resolve itself. The day Maria was set to move home was the same day my otherwise reliable husband, slipped off the roof and broke his foot.

As I awaited Maria's return to her home, I received a call from Lincoln in the E.R. He would be undergoing foot surgery and expected to be bedridden for 6 weeks or more. I would be his main nurse during this period. The timing of the incident could not have been worse, as the 24-hour cycle of caregivers would not be secured for my mother. This triangle of my husband's needs and Maria's needs would continue to plague me for the next two and a half years or so. Some days, as I drove down the central boulevard that ran between my parents' house and my family's house, I would not know what direction to turn, Maria's house or home? I was always torn between the two.

April

April, always by Kurt's side, was much like a Wagnerian beauty, with a strong build and physical aptitude. She was often found sitting on the sofa next to Kurt, holding his hand.

"You love me, don't you?" he would say, and then he would ask; "You are one of my people, aren't you? Or " Darling let's go away together."

All this happened under my mother's watchful eye. I knew she understood that his mind had slipped away, but did his devotions to April really upset her? I think not, as she was above most of what happened around her.

Laura

Laura was my mother's special assistant. She was a single mother of a very lovely and pale Goth young woman, who would also spend time with Maria having tea. I was always impressed with Maria's ability to accept all kinds of people in a non-judgmental way. Imagine an elderly proper Victorian woman, chitchatting with a young free spirit with plum hair band lots of piercings and leather. Laura, with her bulldog-stance and hard edge mannerisms, ripe with sarcasm and wit, had a chip on her shoulder about men and their ability to take women on rides in life. Her cynical edge was always softened by Maria's charm. Laura was a true guardian of Maria, and growled furiously if anyone upset her cares, emotionally or physically. My mother embraced her dotage and relied on her fiercely.

Vladamina

Vladamina was an unusual caregiver who moved to La Crosse to be with her Bulgarian daughter from Greece. She must have been Bulgarian too and eager for work, with little knowledge of English. She would say, "I do it," about everything we needed, including the more difficult hoyer lift. I would see them spending hours trying to manage that device, with Maria hanging in limbo, looking like a small child on a swing. After Vladamina mastered the delicate positioning of Maria and the lift, she suddenly did not show one day as we were told that she had to return to Greece to care for another elderly lady. Maria was really left hanging then.

Rebecca

Rebecca was a strong, youthful, and vivacious brunette who always wore pink and insisted that Maria was dressed in pink at all times. Pink had never been Maria's favorite color and this was especially annoying. They behaved like Princesses together. She was writing a romance novel on the side and she would entertain Maria with this story for hours.

Marilyn

Marilyn was mostly the errand-runner, giving Kurt rides and getting groceries. She was also the house-cleaner. She was an attractive blond woman who spent winters in Florida, but kept a place in La Crosse, as well, despite on old hubby who stayed back. She had spent her life raising a family and running the kids' rides at the local park with her husband. She kept a pet pigeon and many cats. She was a regular and easygoing presence in the house.

Jane

Jane was there towards the end. She had reassured me before I left for a long weekend with my husband, that Maria would be there when I returned.

She was an attractive and bubbly and fair lady with a love of the elderly and cats. She swooned over Kurt and Maria's white cat Moony, (the one that Kurt threw across the room when he had fits of rage). Moony would always return to his side, for more. Her last report to me was that she and Dan barely got Maria out of bed on her final day of living, that wintry day in early February of 2007.

Jane was also the pain pill counter, and she would call me in a panic that four pain pills or so were missing. Sometimes I thought Maria forgot that she took them, as she was on a regimen of as many as eight pills a day for her debilitating rheumatic pain, which never seems to have fully burned out.

Often, Jane would accuse Dan of stashing some away in his very, very messy downstairs abode. One day, I was sent down there with Jane to inspect, and I found mounds of dirty clothes and food, strange health vitamins and devices (like his chi machine), to trip over and sort through. I found everything one could imagine in that basement bedroom, but the missing pain pills, (which, according to Jane and April could be sold for a pretty penny on the open market.)

Later, I read in the newspaper that Jane was on probation for stealing pain pills at an elderly clients home. I then understood where all the "pill anxiety" came from in Maria's house, but I never suspected her, due to her keen devotion to Maria and the cat.

Juan and Berta

Juan and Berta was a Colombian couple that cared for Maria alone in the end. Their adventures with us deserve a chapter to themselves.

8

*L*ast week, I agreed to take Kurt to see the geriatric specialist to have his medications checked. He had been frequently agitated and difficult to handle so we as caregivers hoped an adjustment in the Lorazepam schedule would resolve some of the difficulty. As I left Kurt in a sunny quadrant of the lobby, while I parked my car—I noticed a distinguished middle-aged man sitting in the corner waiting. Somehow I intuited that he was focused on us. When I returned, he was questioning my father and abruptly asked me, "Are you Joan Gundersen? —Is this Mr. Happe, I presume? I need to speak with you alone. I am Bill Johnson of the County Health—Aging Department and I'm here to take custody of him for a 72-hour observation period. You see Mr. Happe is a danger to himself and the community."

I was completely dumbfounded. My gut previously had told me something was brewing but this was almost surreal, or should I say alarmingly real.

"Nobody is taking my father anywhere. He is agitated and angry at the time and this is why I'm taking him to his doctor to get his meds adjusted. He lives in a loving home with his wife, whose sole purpose these days is caring for her husband. My main career is Kurt. He is just as dangerous in a nursing home situation. He could fall there too. He no longer wanders. This is ridiculous."

I could see that this county officer had been put in his place!

"Well take care of him and see that there are no more complaints about him. The neighbors care for his safety, and call me if needed."

I wasn't quite sure what to make of this Mr. Johnson. Was he a friend or foe?

A day later, once the excitement had passed, I found Kurt reacting well to his new medicine trial. He and his second beloved cat, Gabby (who looks as he is dressed in a tuxedo,) was enjoying moments of sunshine together. I gave him a hug and told them they were both very loved and adorable.

"And who am I to you?" he asked.

"I am your beloved daughter of 43 years!"

"Oh really," he replied and yet somehow seemed very satisfied, and I as his personal advocate also took great satisfaction.

Somehow, as a caregivers we felt between a rock and a hard place. If we asked for a new RN on his homecare case it could impact the homecare staff already in transition and Kurt could be discharged. Then we would find ourselves out in the cold or back at point A. If we called a patient rights' advocate a case would be made and our county officer would be accused. Would that be helpful? If we called the Aging Resources Center and got the county officer; all calls would be referred to him again as I had already once experienced. So back to just not making waves and trying to survive.

Here is a poem Lili (Kurt's granddaughter) wrote about her grandpa around this time,

By Lili, age 16

Kurt:

He stamps his cane and claps his hands—

always precisely to the beat

but I cannot hear the music.

Sometimes he cries

Because the song is so beautiful

and I wish I could cry with him.

"Be quiet," he will tell me.

"Can't we just listen?"

I always try, but it's never there.

Sometimes he asks me what I am to him.

Your granddaughter, I reply with a kiss

and I want to cry because he is so beautiful.

He may not remember my name but

he still has his rhythm.

9

My sister Marina, who visited frequently from Baltimore and would do whirlwind tours of organizing 330 S. 21st. street when she came, was a wonderful support and resource for our parents care, even though the distance prevented her from being on the front-line. Although we did not always agree on the best care strategy, she offered all of us her moral support and home organizational skills, filling the house with supplies for winter and ways to improve Kurt and Maria's lifestyle in their home. Here is a letter she wrote me about care resources for our father:

Dear Joanie, I would love to design Mom's invitation. What are your ideas for a celebration for Dad's 80th birthday party? Or maybe if Dad is settled in a nursing home, you could bring Mom to DC this spring? Regarding the county person, I do think you should identify where they were planning on taking Dad that day.

I have been reading a great book at the library, " Alzheimer's, A Caregiver's Guide and Sourcebook" by Howard Kreutzer. He makes a great point that although the caregiver may want to keep the loved one at home, and institution may be the only realistic alternative. Did you know that falling might mean that Dad may have forgotten to walk and should be checked for a stroke? On pg. 32, it says that the end of life will most likely be drawn out with difficulty breathing, eating, choking and even coma. This will be so impossible for Mom and all of us. Let's think about this before the need becomes critical. Let's decide about a Nursing home or Hospice care at home. Also he warns that stress for a caregiver is likely to grow and we must watch for signs of depression.   He says that grief is hidden by the demands of care giving but there must be time for ongoing mourning. My thoughts are that putting Dad in a home, will take away Mom's main role in her life, so that is why she resists and we must reinforce to her that her role is important as ever when she finally will get quality time for visiting Dad at the care center. The book made me ask myself "Can Dad's total needs be provided for on a 24 hour basis? Will mom's stamina severely be taxed by Dad's needs? Will Mom's health concerns begin to rival Dad's? What do the Physicians suggest? Can Mom still really handle all this? Her feelings of guilt may apparently make her be unclear about the ability to accept the problems in caring for her husband. I hope this is helpful! Love, Marina

* 10 *

Even though on many visits to see my father, I would find him very agitated or in an altered apathetic state on his living room sofa; it would have been easy to turn away from him and close off our relations; leave him all to the paid caregivers. I never really entertained this thought—only once when his anger was so very great and he hit me rather strongly with his cane. I felt the ache in my knee and I was also reminded of a heart-ache that I think I always carried with me, that of the un-validated and somewhat verbally abused eldest daughter; a wound that I carried from childhood. Even as I try to recollect this phase of my upbringing, I begin to slump over on my writing desk. My father's regular belittling of me was then mostly around my inability to comprehend elementary school math as a young girl. He was an engineering whiz, a graduate of MIT and he did not do well with my shortcoming. 'Maria, how can she be so stupid,' he would say, and words of that nature. Later I came to realize that his coolness towards us at times stemmed from his being an only child in Germany and from being left behind by his parents at the age of two and a half, so that they could find a new life in America. He did not join them until he was 16 and he carried the temperament of an isolated, wounded child with him throughout life.

Mostly I would find humor in his odd behaviors. One time he was found running around in his underwear at the disapproval of his caregiver Ellen Schmidt who had a way of dealing with his odd behaviors. I assume he monsterized her and in his mind she was a dark controlling force. He hated always to be told what to do. Ellen was able to ignore the grimace that he would make as he haunted her behind her back, following her from room to room. I chose to return to his side in these last years of his decline because I felt a feeling of satisfaction in finally having him physically present there with my mother.

For the years of my childhood, my father was often vague in his physical presence, either traveling in the Mideast or with his thoughts beyond our own in the esoteric world of geopolitics. During his Alzheimer's condition he finally became present for me, really there with me.

Today I slip in the back porch and listen a bit; I would often do this to catch the reality of their home-life and the passing temperaments. How did they function when I was not there to lean on? Were they really in a precarious situation? Today I notice the porch is covered with small plastic cups of a cider-colored drink. Is this urine or cider? When I enter I see the large green bottle of cherry wine Maria has been concocting. It is an old recipe of fermented cherries, which will turn into a delicious summer wine they tell me; yet I notice there is a layer of gnats or fruit flies in the bottle too. 'Does she not see this, I wonder…. won't drinking gnats make her ill?

"Oh it's fine, it won't hurt it. You'll see. It will be delicious. We can drink it on the deck."

Maria's beautiful deck garden, filled with potted flowers, was her link to beauty, peace and sanctity. She would often sit there in the afternoon, just feeling the warmth of the sun on her ragged joints. This gave her great pleasure.

One of my favorite pastimes was giving Kurt rides in the car. Not only did it give Maria a necessary breather, he loved it. Often when we returned to 330 S. 21st street, Kurt refused to get out of the car and I had to really coax him out. He would often be the most complementary on these trips and would tell me that I had such fine driving skills. He had had his own driver in Italy, where he worked, as an engineer, Mario Martinelli. He would always tell him to slow down in Italian—'piano, piano,' he would direct. He would also use this same phrase if I went over 40 in a neighborhood zone. 'By the way,' he would say, 'do you have your running lights on?'—This was his biggest concern that we would be driving without headlights.

"I feel a neblina."

"What's that dad?"

"A fog. It is very foggy out."

He would see all in a mist despite that it was a bright and clear day, due to his macular degeneration. I would always reassure him; yes I do have my running lights. Don't worry! Always we would go for drives up Bliss road, passed the tacky German style Alpine Inn and onwards to the scenic rural landscape of the Mississippi bluff land. When we ran out of conversation he would tap his cane and chant, "Bingo, Bango, Bongo. That's the way it is in the Congo," as his past days of travel also took him into deep and dark parts of Africa.

I would often find messages lying around the house – notes of overnight happenings. There were many of these little communication notes left around between caregivers. Some were amusing. Here are a few:

January 25th

Friday eve–

I got in around 11:30pm. Kurt still up, pounding. Maria asleep. The white noise machine is great!

I went up and asked Kurt to stop pounding. I think it had some effect.

I took a bath and fell asleep to waterfalls.

Love you Joanie,

Joy

In addition, my sister created this handwritten flow chart detailing their daily care needs. It was much like an elaborate jigsaw puzzle to fill in the spaces. (See Weekly Care Schedule on page 36) and April's notes:

The most effective way to deal with Kurt is:

If sleeping pat him softly and quietly say his name. If he is startled he gets angry.

Whisper in his ear as to what you want him to do. This is more effective than repeating things when he says, "What?"

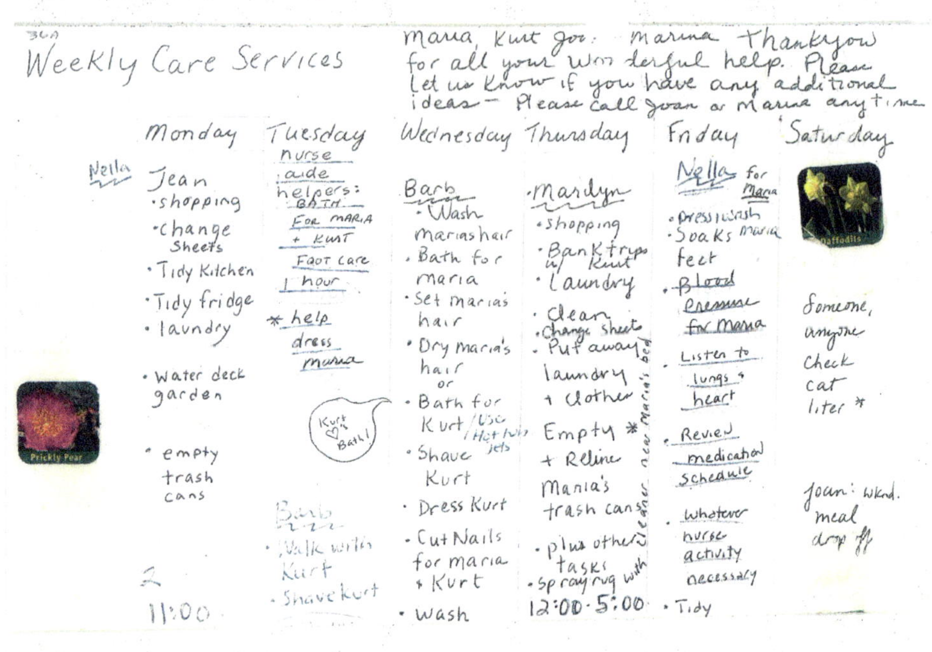

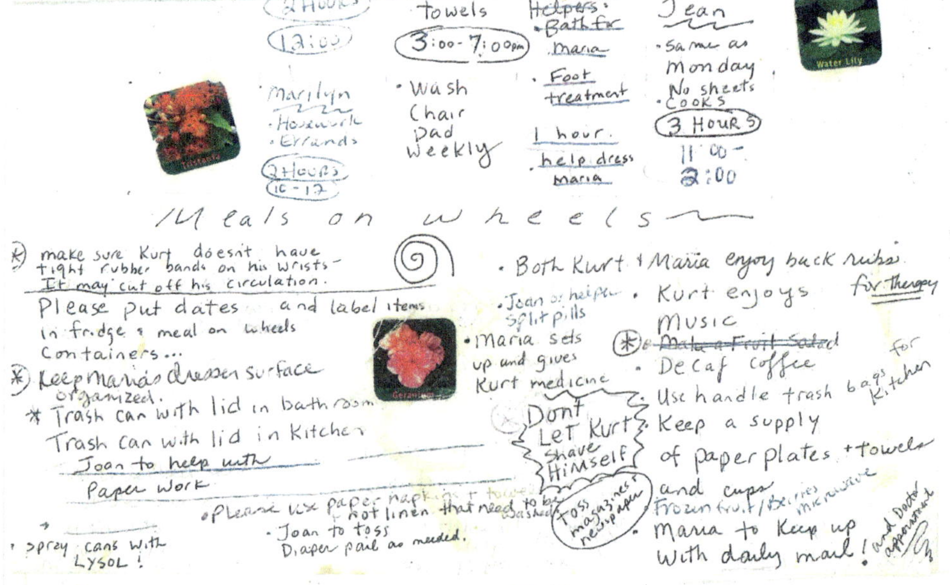

Marina created this weekly flow chart to organize their care

If angry, try affection. Example: "Can I have a hug?" or, pat his arm and tell him you understand.

Ignore any directions to go to hell as he sends us there daily.

Don't treat him like a child!!!!! He is very smart and doesn't understand what is happening to him.

Report any odd things to Mrs. Happe, as it is her right to know first. She is his Power of Attorney.

Don't force his cares if he says NO. It is ok to try waiting 5 minutes or try a different task first. If he still resists, don't worry about it. April will try later that day.

If Kurt is confrontational just talk to him and he will follow you.

If not, oh well these are the stages of Alzheimer's and they will pass. We can't change things but we do our best to make his days the best for him. We all have bad days, we can handle them, but Kurt doesn't know what's happening to him and we need to be understanding and sympathetic to him.

This evening when I fix the broken bulb on their bedroom fan lamp, Kurt comes up from behind me and socks me in the lower back. I am caught off guard for he now sees me as an intruder. I hear Maria scolding him, 'Kurt, this is our daughter.' It is a triple pain for me: 1) The reminder of childhood hurt 2) The physical pain of his hit on my back 3) The present pain in the knowledge, that he "does not know who I really am." When I shared his rude behavior with an old family friend she said, "just let him pass," but there is still his cute and lovable side, I tell her, so this is not an easy solution either.

Sometimes I felt that the reason my father has become what he is, often ridiculous with outrageous behaviors is to be a foil to all our foolish societal conventions. Yesterday, when my mother, myself and our Mexican friend Violeta were having one of our regular teas together; Maria's favorite past-time, Violeta was sharing about an upcoming trip to Mexico and sipping tea when we notice Kurt frantically unzipping his pants and holding a tea cup with painted roses right up to his fly. We think he is ready to pee into one of Maria's lovely teacups! I quickly suggest we go to the men's room instead. I had placed a line of neon-colored tape on the floor as a guide to tell him to follow the path. "Cie la vie;" or 'Chacun son goût' each to his own desires –Kurt is following his own motto for living.

I have thoughts of Kurt as a burgermeister, a more rough German personality trying to fit into my mother's aristocratic world, the world of lady-in-waitings and empresses; yet instead of the expected behavior of a high society lady snubbing him, she behaved like a true blueblood, very accepting of all and only lifting an eyebrow at his base behavior. While my mother's indomitable spirit is evident, I see in her eyes that she is tired and it is only a matter of time before she will give up. My consoling effort is to let Kurt live in a retirement home, but she reminds me that he still knows enough to tell her he loves her "in the dark of the night." She is strong spirited, but also must break as we all do. She goes on to tell me that last night he came very close to her to ask some pressing questions, "Who am I? And why am I here?" She very patiently explains but has to laugh when he asks her, "Are you male or female? What is your relationship to me?" "I'm your wife," she says. "Oh, I see. That's nice," He replies. Their bond has always been one of love.

Lately, Kurt has taken up a new hobby to get through the night. He has begun to tap his cane in full force. I call him, "Mr. Tappy;" instead of "Mr. Happe." We wish there was a band he could join to express his new passion. He taps complicated rhythms to the classical music station and gets very angry with anyone who tries to silence him. "Bravo Maestro! Bravo! Bravo!" He seems so joyful tapping and clapping. Kurt yells, "Go to hell!" Maria responds with a smile and says, "Show me the way." Mother reminds us all with her uplifting words, "Make the best of life's circumstances as things turn out in mysterious ways."

Kurt's incontinence continues to get progressively worse; the wet sofa in the living room, a family antique from Philadelphia days is covered in newspapers. The house has a definite urine stench. I wonder how to manage the cleanliness of the place. Laura, the devoted helper yells, "Febreeze it and put it out back." Maybe it really is time for them to go to the care center? They goal was to keep them in their own home until they are both beyond repair. I do believe Kurt is already beyond care center qualifications.

Sometimes when I felt depleted and overwhelmed I would repeat this prayer to myself:

> Let nothing disturb thee...
> Nothing affront thee.
> All things are passing.
> God never changeth.
> Patience, endurance
> Attaineth to all things
> Who God possesseth
> In nothing wanting...
> Alone God sufficeth.

> — St. Theresa of Avila

In my reading I came across these suggested lifestyle changes for caregivers:

— Get adequate sleep
— Healthy diet is paramount
— Exercise regularly for fitness and stress relief
— Schedule your regular health check-up
— No alcohol abuse!
— Schedule time with family and friends
— Nurse your own interests
— Be kind to yourself– love, honor, and value yourself
— Educate yourself about your loved one's condition. Information is empowering.
— Seek support from other caregivers. There is great strength in knowing that you are not alone...

* 11 *

More and more I come to realize that I am overly reactive and issues are there to experience, to exist with, but not necessarily to be dealt with. I also come to terms with the fact that I cannot be all things to all people but need to maintain a path of my very own. Baba calls this way "selfish" but it is really only a mode of survival without becoming ill; sickness may be a manifestation of being lost from one's own path, although I was innately certain that caring and loving them, as their dutiful and eldest daughter was a segment of this path.

As Maria's bedsores became deadly and unmanageable and Kurt is getting into more and more fiasco's at home, it is clear, that at least Kurt must head off to a care center. Maria cannot be without him it seems, and insists on joining him. We are all in need of respite of sorts. My parents can both be managed for a bit, or maybe it will be a permanent solution. They are assigned to a small double room at the end of a sunny hall of a medical unit where they will be cared for and monitored around the clock. Maybe Maria's bedsores will finally heal. She is given an air mattress to circulate air and heal her sores. I can finally feel at ease that they are being cared for, and that Kurt will endanger himself less.

My family is given the opportunity to stay in an old beach house in Cape-Cod for a few days and we leap at the chance for a change of scene. Resettling Kurt and Maria away from their cozy place has been stressful. I don't miss the in-house conflict that had arisen between their caregivers. April and Paddhie are ready to have a real blowout

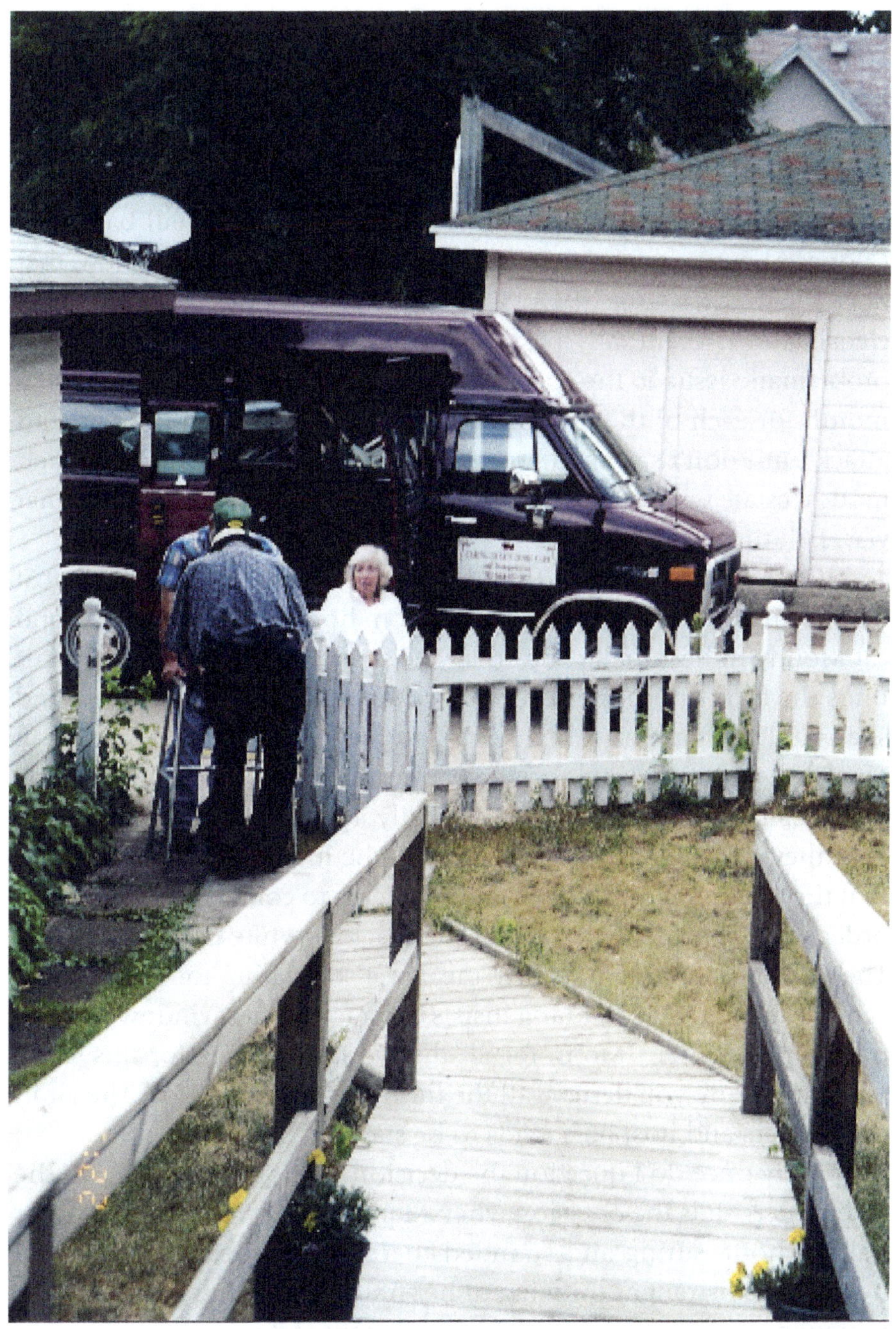

Kurt and Maria going to the Care Center to live

fist fight in the backyard. There is clearly an issue of clashing person-alities. Paddhie complains about Marilyn's inability to clean well.

"Rugs should be washed, not just air-dried," Paddhie insists. Marilyn simply rolls her eyes when I mention anything to do with Paddhie.

I am also showing signs of wear and tear. The small bald spot (alopecia) has increased from the size of a dime to a quarter now, that doctor says. I had one at 18 years of age after a bout with mononu-cleosis and it eventually passed, so I disregard it for now. Another problematic issue is the cost of care for my parents, about $3,500 a month for each of them. I think the bill will give them both a heart attack but I don't see an alternate for any of us. At this amount their modest estate will be depleted. Although I don't think there is another way. Full time care costs!

Over time we all get used to this new scenario. I visit almost daily, bringing them treats and items from home including the second cat Moony in her small cat carrier. The staff is very attentive and Kurt finds the food appealing. Maria likes the new bath system there and she is able to have a real bath instead of the at home sponge bath. They find new acquaintances there and strong and able young people to transfer them and help them in daily activities. The staff wonders how they ever managed on their own. The lunches are so nutritious that they both put on a few pounds. I decide to come once a week and order a tray to share with them in the spacious white recreation room. The balanced, sit-down, hearty meal is also healing for me. Despite care center regulations, Maria insists on cracking her window to let in fresh air. I tell her, "Mom, for all that you are paying for this small cramped room, you deserve all the fresh air that you need." The air in care centers and hospitals tends to be stagnant.

Only once do I question the decision to have them reside in the care center—it is the occasion when Maria is left on the toilet for over half an hour, sitting and stranded there despite her many calls for help. I was distraught thinking of her frail body sitting there and for-gotten in this very uncomfortable, indignant state.

We spend many wonderful evenings sitting together out on the patio surrounded by the summer flowers and warm summer air. Kurt no longer says much, but looks well with his weathered olive skin, summer "cappy" and cotton madras print shirts. On one occasion he came very close to me in his chair and cupped both my knees. He held his hands there for some time and somehow this action seemed to complete me and to say our earthly cycle as father and daughter was soon to come to a close. I felt myself strengthen at this time as if some kind of spiritual transference was occurring between he and I. There were other signs that things were ending—Paddhie who was still residing in the house as a caretaker of the home, cat and plants—had turned his large portrait of himself in an American Officer suit around so it faced the wall. Strangely closer to the day of his death, before she knew he had left this place, it had disappeared all together. I was ready to report it to the police, but it was found in the attic in a dusty corner. I had been having nightmares of his passing in a metaphorical sense—images of large black Hearst-like cars arriving at his 21st street address to take him away. In any case, I realized I had lost him over the years in bits and pieces. This was only saying goodbye to the shell of the man, ravaged by Alzheimers and dementia, who had been my father.

Kurt's Farewell

Today, at 4pm, on the regular tea visit, I am surprised to find Kurt in bed, fully dressed with shallow breathing. The skin on his face falls tightly back and away on his skull- almost taunt but not vital. Is this what a death mask looks like, I wonder? I try not to look too long but the artist in me wants to draw him. My other forces tell me to look away. Here is the drawing I quickly rendered at his side. Since he hardly speaks anymore, I wonder what he knows, what he experiences. Often, I find him sitting in a chair with a heavy head dropped down over his diminished but still heavy build. The weight of his presence is great and burdensome. Soon after this, his breath changed, and his labs went haywire. Kurt left rather quietly and peacefully. His breathing shallow from his diaphragm, his mouth gaped open and recalled his more sedentary lifestyle at the center probably, signs of death. I was able to see him in this state, and I told him I'd see him in the morning. The CNA on duty <u>promised</u> me that my father would survive. I squeezed his hand and he seemed semi-conscious.

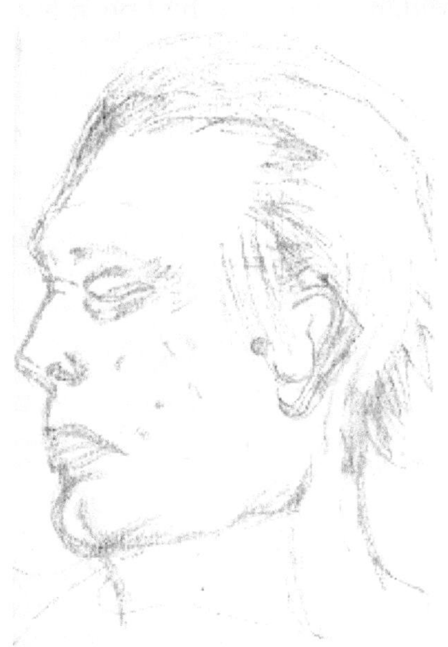

Drawing of Kurt at the end.

My daughter, Lili, tells him she loves him, yet he leaves before we can do much else, as if he didn't need to see me again and deal with a long, drawn out ordeal. I sit with his pale body. We drape a scarf over it and give him an icon to hold. Lincoln, and his brother Ralph take him away in Lincoln's old truck, a family tradition of sorts in the Gundersen medical family. It took me a while to accept this practice, but it does save on funeral costs. I take a few photos and touch his arm. His skin is paper-thin. I was informed at 7a.m. that day, that dad leaves this world. Dad told me "alles gut, endes gut" – all is well that ends well. His quiet ending to a long and rich life filled with travel, friends, loving family and good food made it all for the best. His last phase was just hanging on at thousands per month and he was not thriving in this state. If he had gone home, he was an accident waiting to happen. It was for the best, that it happened the way it did.

I felt a heavy heart 2 days before he left; the missing portrait hidden by Paddhie was a sign of things to come. After my father's death, the sky had beautiful airy wisps and a bright orange glowing sun. I do hope his spirit has made its journey. The mysterious winds after his cremation time make me wonder if he did. I did my best for him and I do realize I gave up a tad early. I did do that, let him go, did not hang on, any more. I never prayed for his departure like Baba, but I understand that it's ok; he's gone, "traveling as always."

I had no idea how my mother would take the news. I think I asked a nurse to tell Maria. Tears filled her eyes, and I noticed her posture stiffen and straighten…she transformed into the individual that she was- strong and unified in herself. We all prayed together. She had realized he was on his way out since his breathing had changed to his mouth from his nose.

On hearing the news, I put on a black flowy skirt, with an oriental design in honor of his love for the exotic and China, which I have never been able to wear since. I rushed to their room at the care center to find the room divider drawn, and Maria on the other side in her sunlit bed, still unaware that Kurt had passed in the night. It broke my heart.

My Mexican friend, Violeta, reassures me, "He is lighter now."

My father was always heavy, so the thought of him finally shedding that weight was comforting. His last year on earth has been a burden and a struggle for everyone involved. We came to believe his struggle would eventually be the means to Baba's own end. I thanked God quietly that she is still here.

In the midst of an in-house gathering of helpers, family, and friends, Paddhie has returned barefoot, and claims she has misplaced her car. I must address the issue of how to cope with her strange behavior and figure out how to get her back on her meds. Yesterday, I found her in the yard picking clovers. This will be the next challenge calling us to live in the midst of our grief. She has been in a sort of angel after all. My mother feels we must let her stay on in the house if only not to disturb her life, but to feed the cat while Maria resides in the center with the hope of healing her severe bedsores. It is clear that all my mother's affairs have become my own now. I hope that I can manage it all.

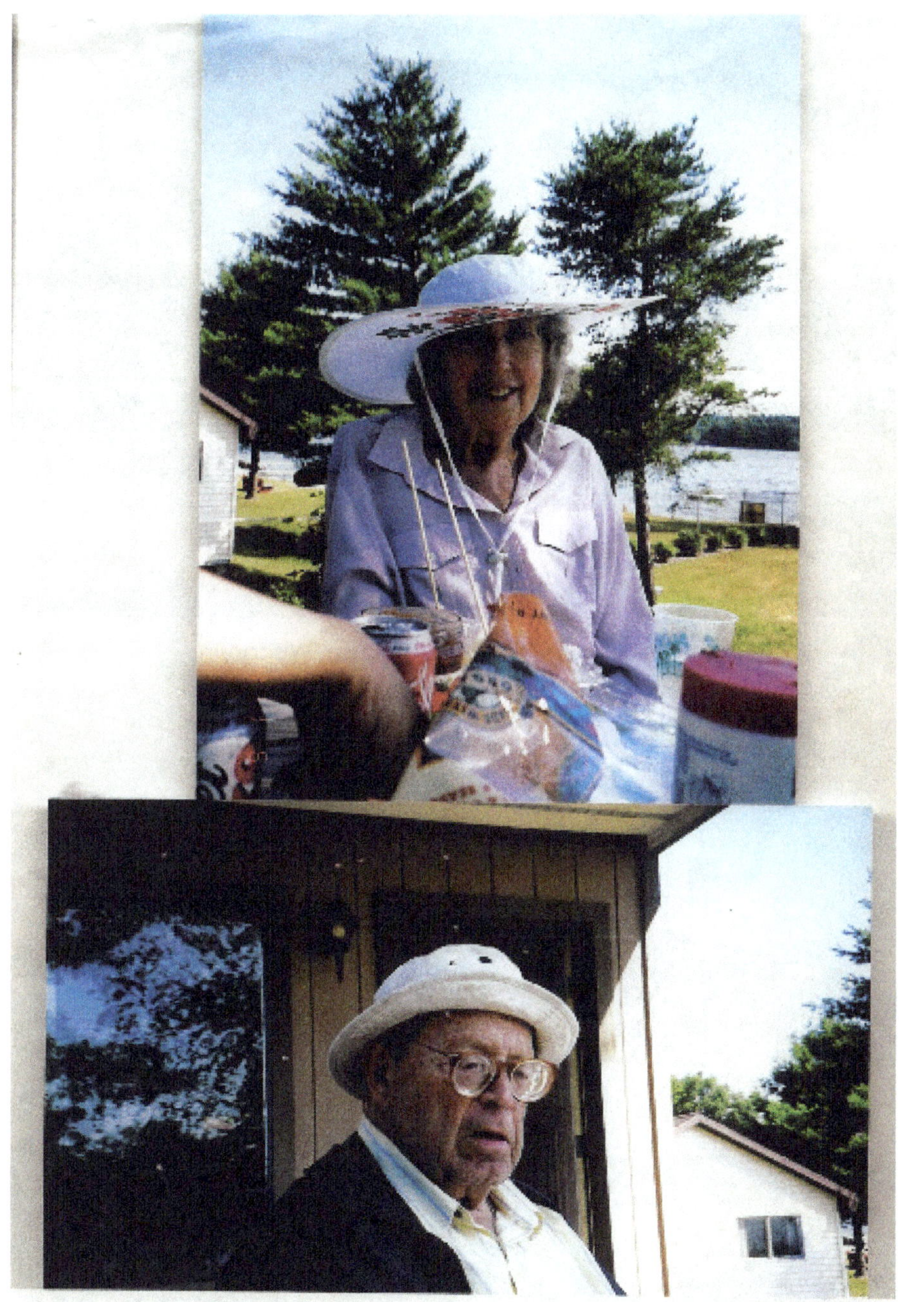

Kurt and Maria at the Dells; Kurt kept us up all night there.

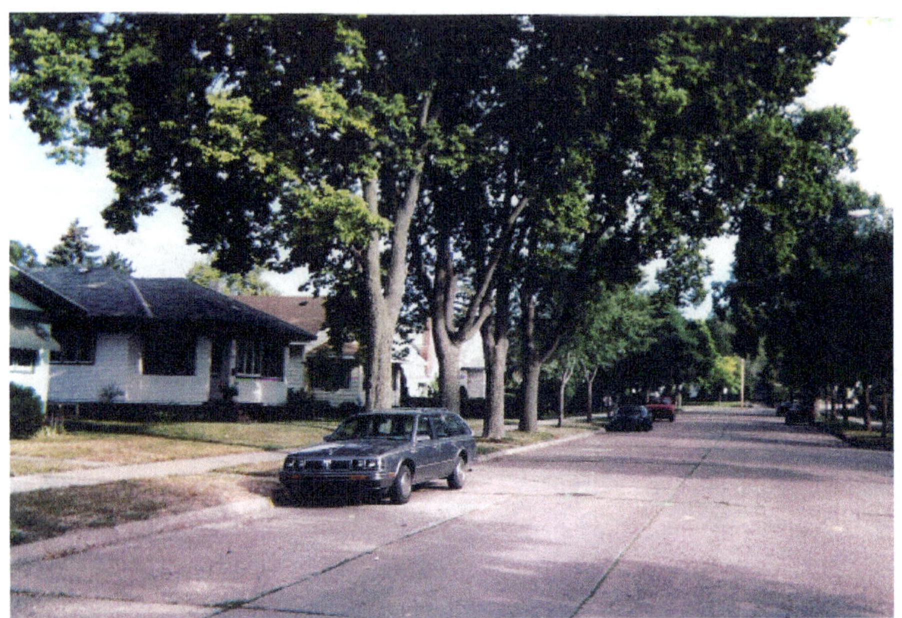

Bungalow at 21st Street, LaCrosse, Wisconsin.

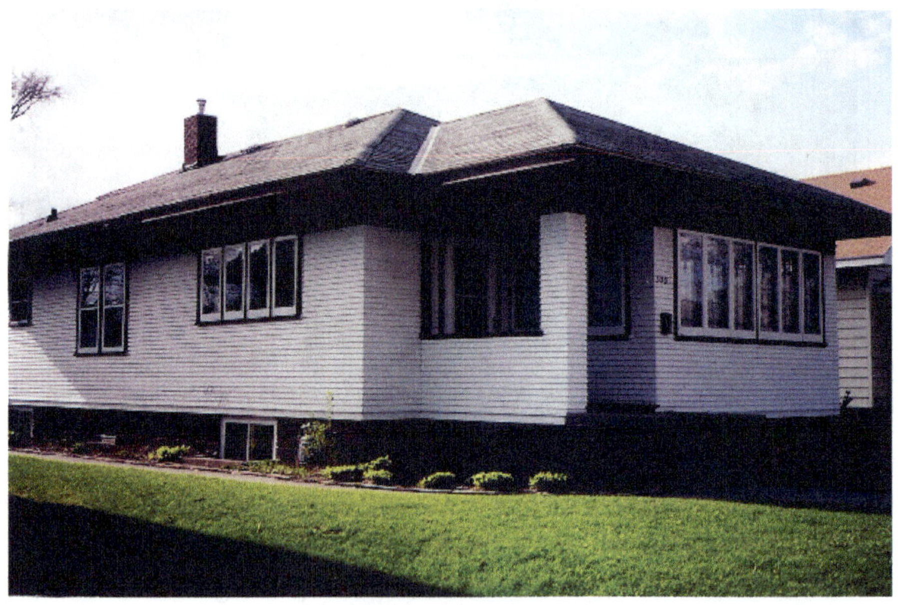

Kurt and Maria's place

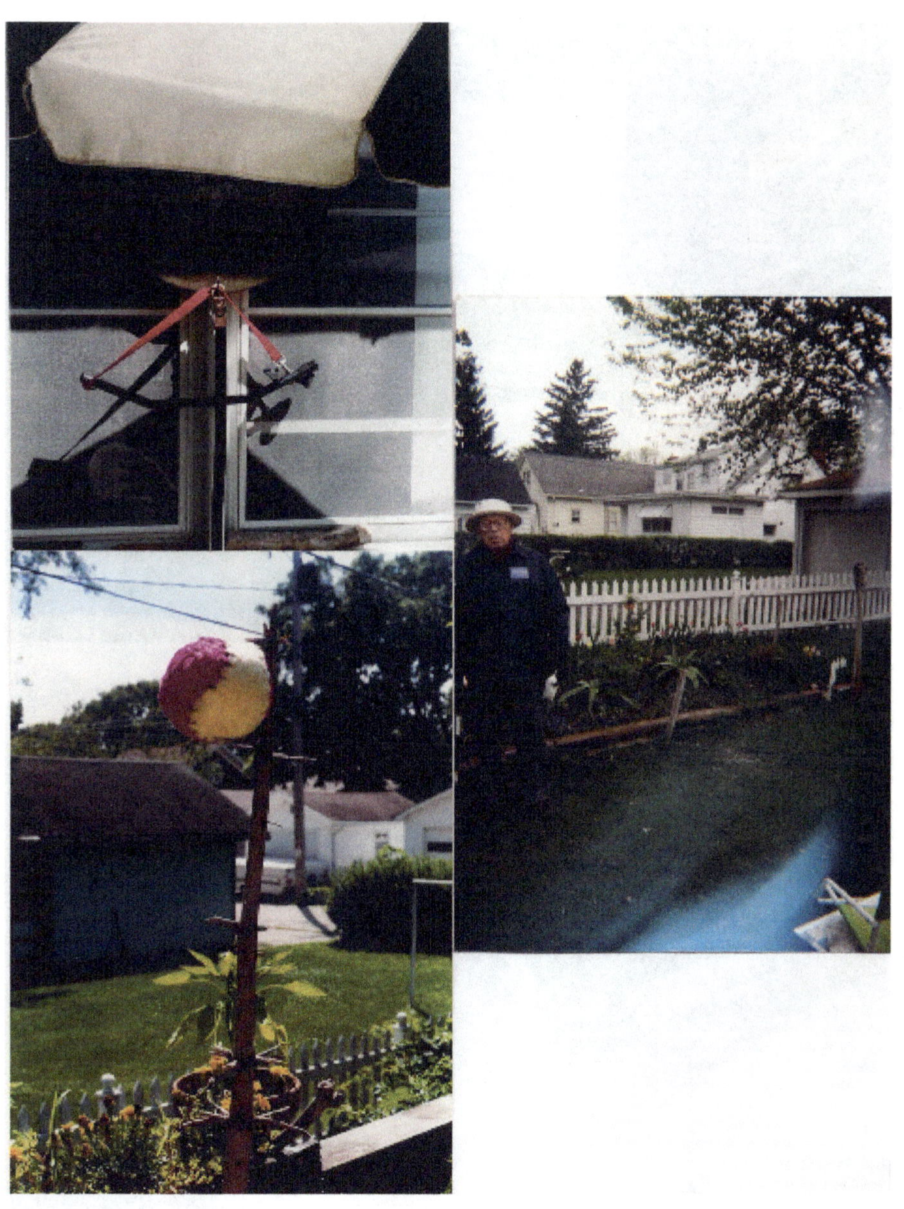

More Yard art Designs by Kurt

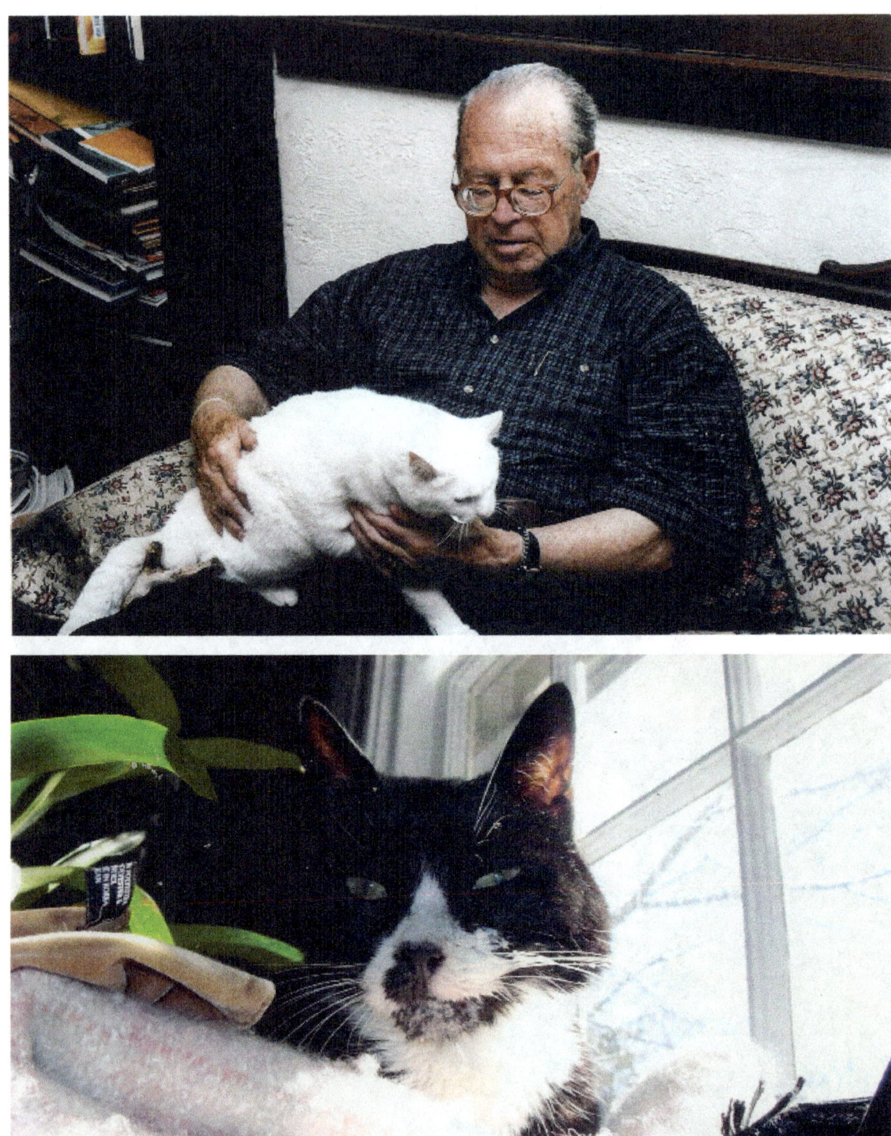

Kurt and his beloved cats; Moony and Gabi

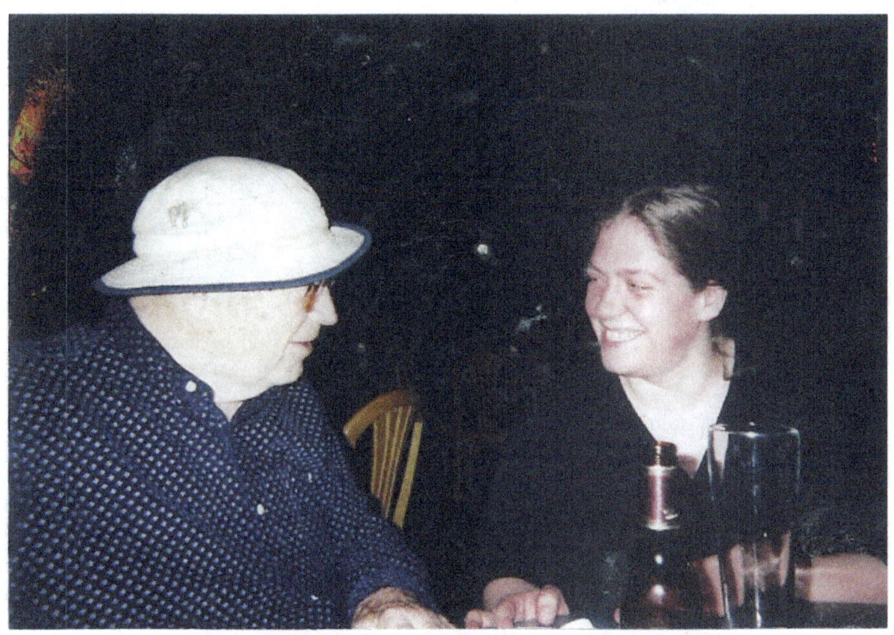

Kurt and Maria with their devoted helpers

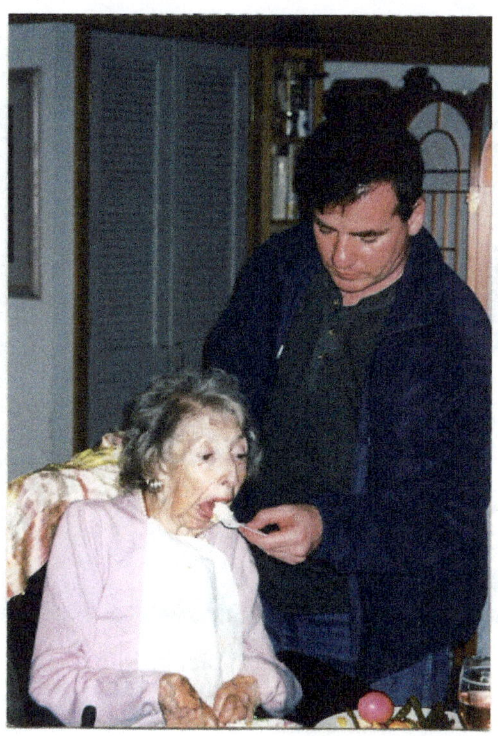

Maria and her caregiver, Dan.

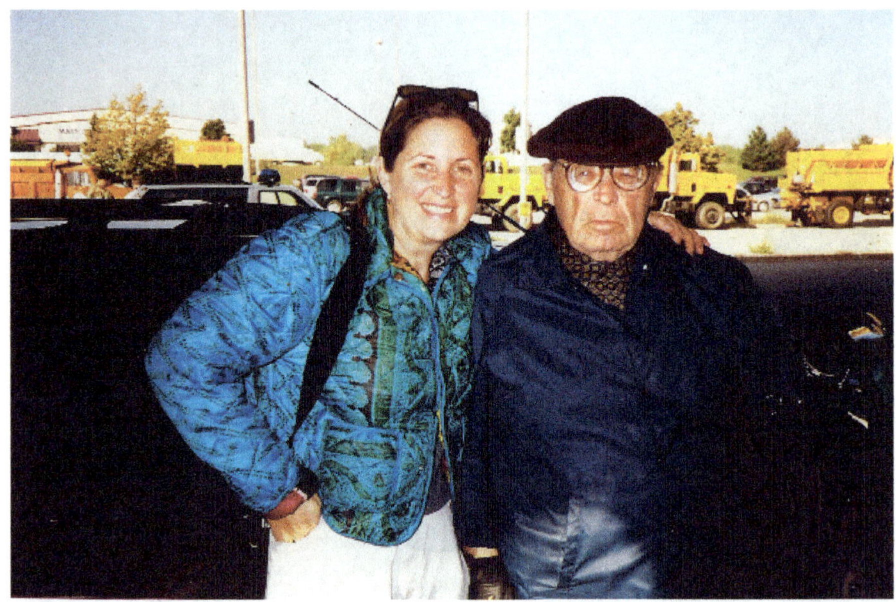

Halcyon days; better times with Kurt and Maria

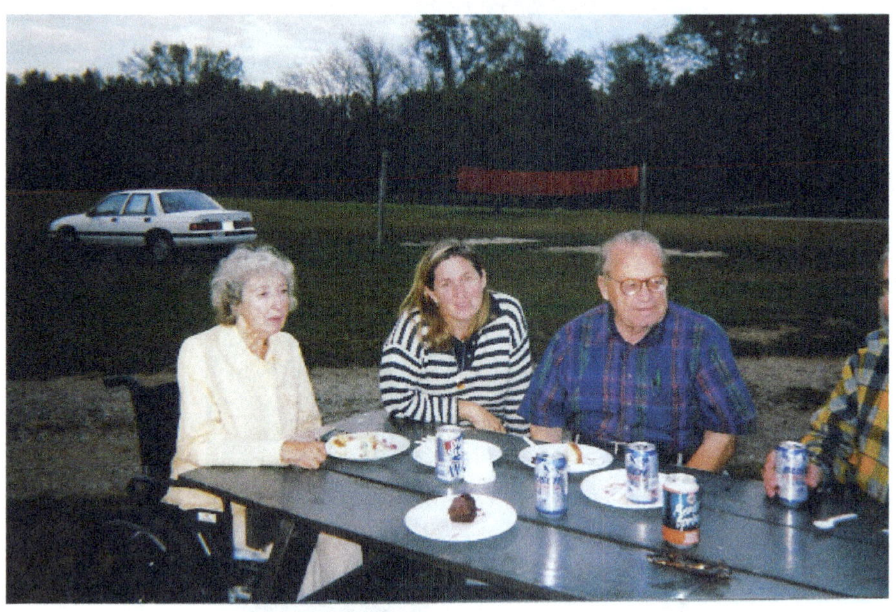

Maria and Kurt at a picnic with me.

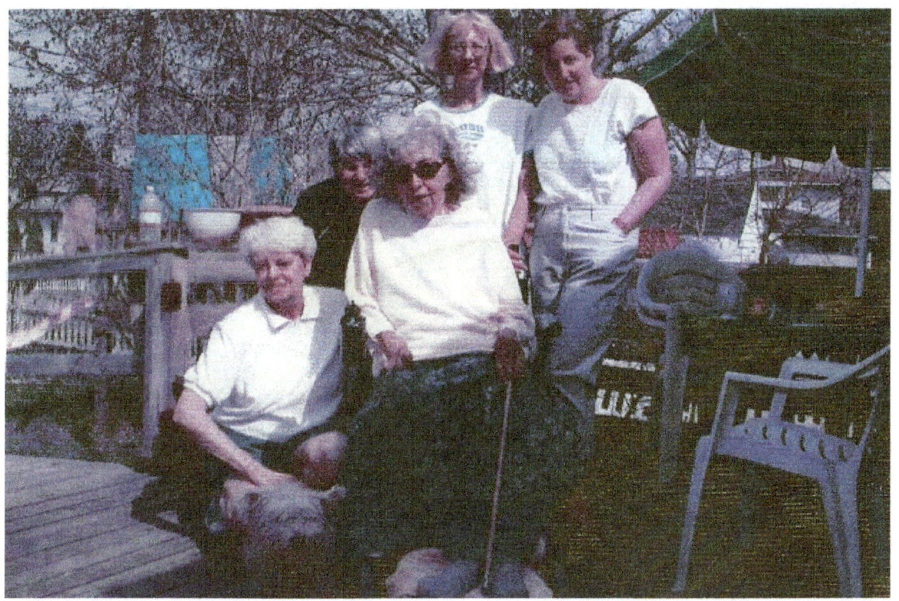

Maria and helpers unite: Marilyn and Paddhie sit to the left of Maria. I am on the far right.

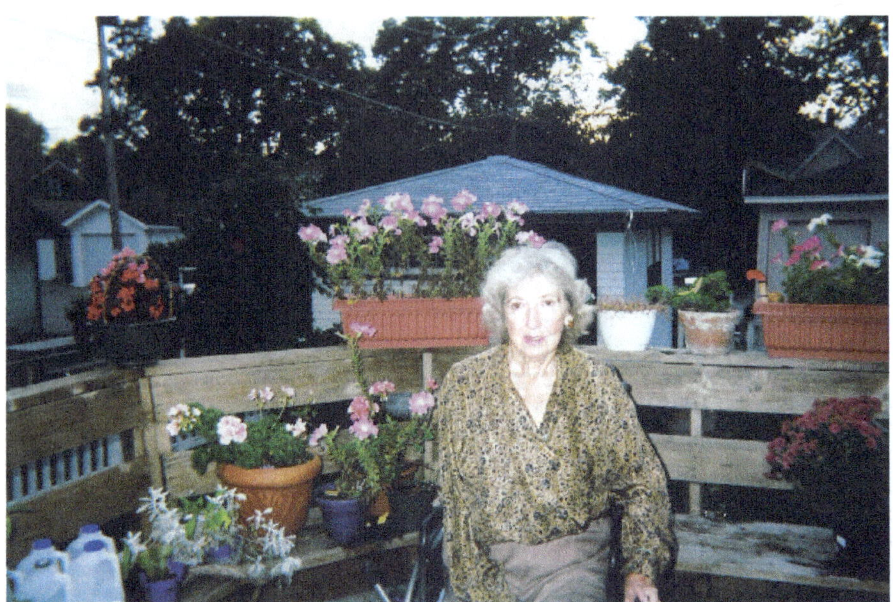

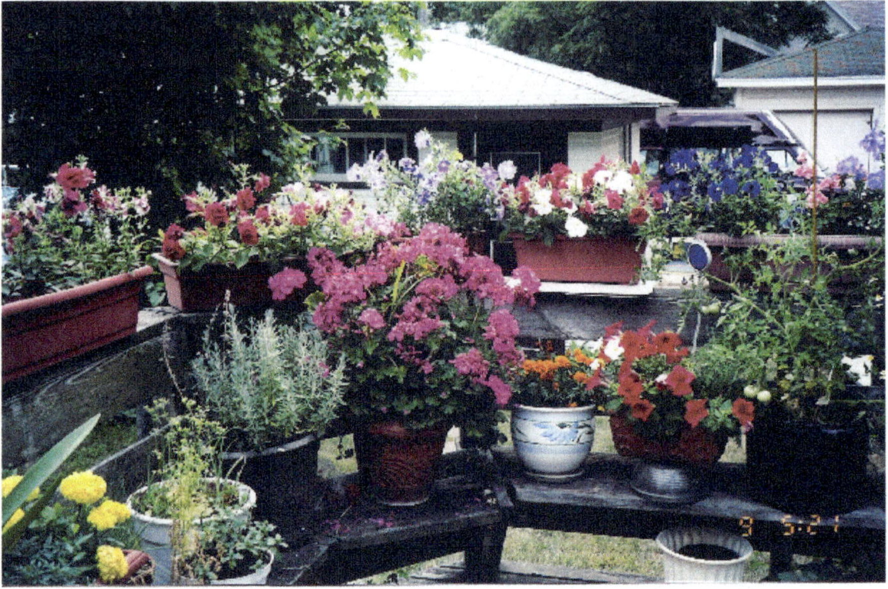

Maria in her deck garden

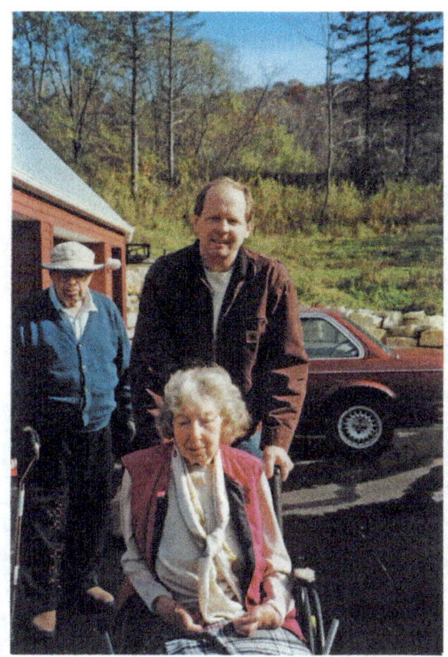

Lincoln with my parents.

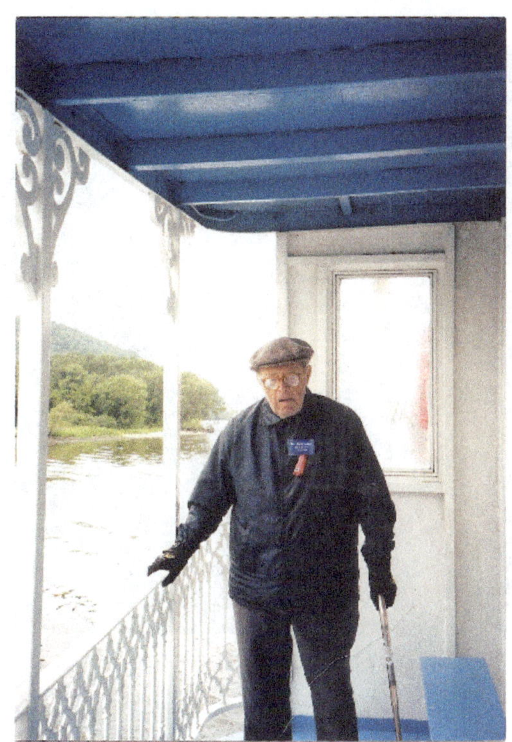

Kurt on a riverboat

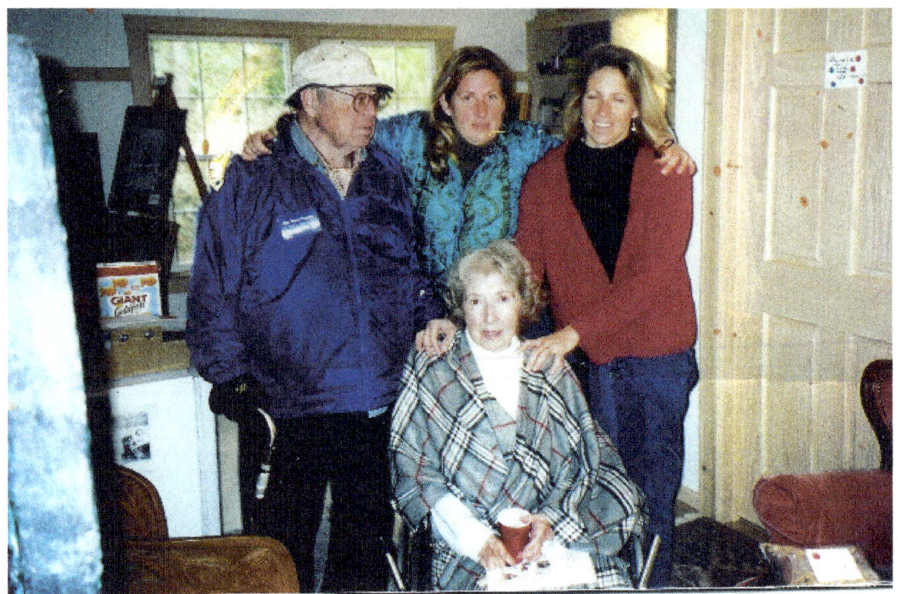

Wisconsin days; Kurt, Joanie, Marina and Maria

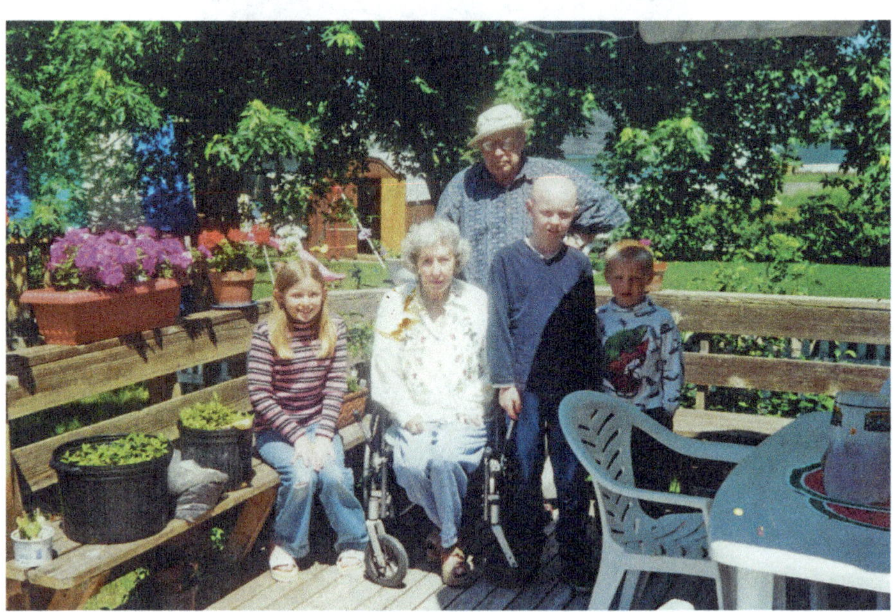

Kurt and Maria with the grand kids.

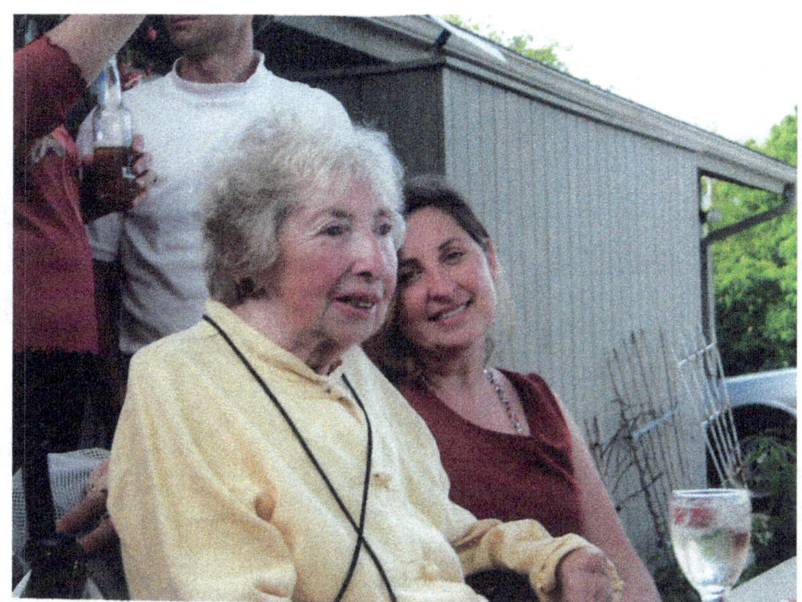

Joan and Maria

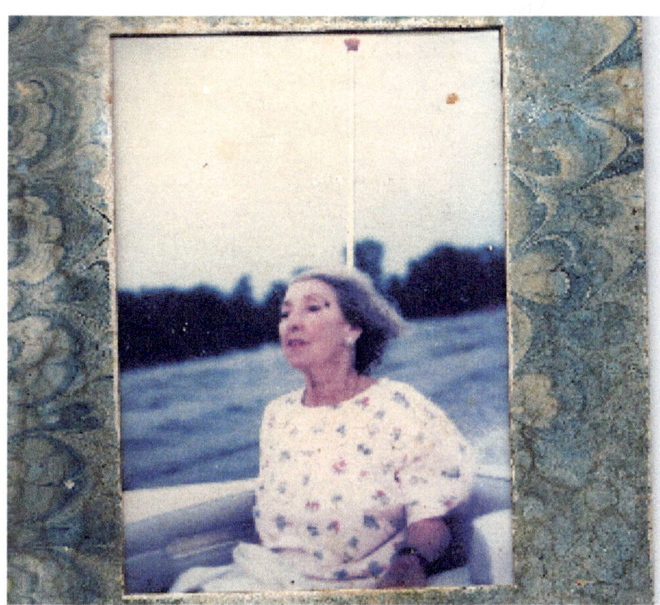

Maria's boat ride captivates her buoyant spirit.

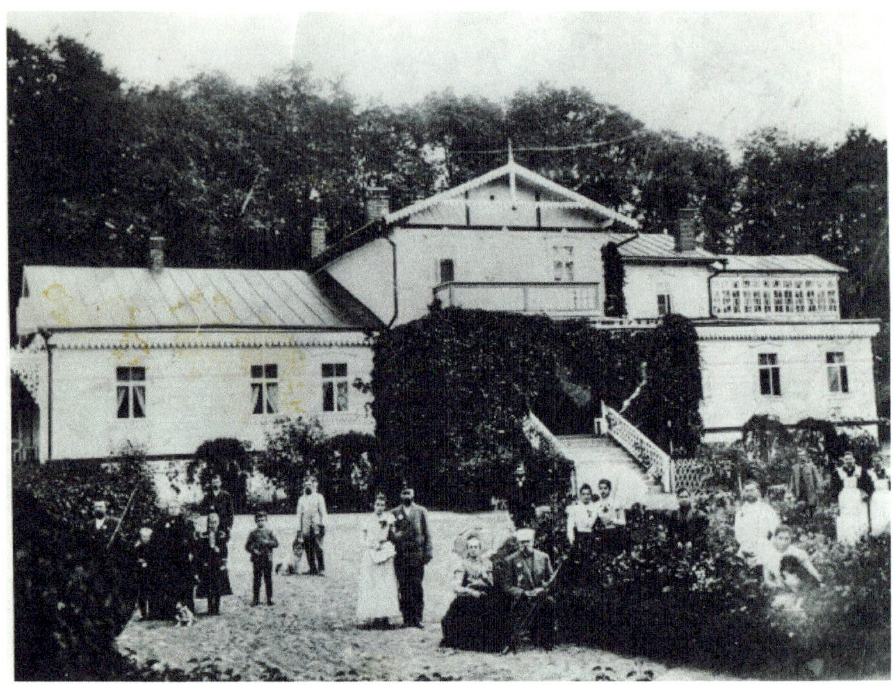

Maria's Poland estate, before WWI.
"Holowiesk"

Borsch - (Ukrainian)
1½ lb. soup meat -
1 lb. fresh pork
½ smoked pork -
10 cups cold water -
1 bay leaf
6 peppercorn
1 bunch soup greens -
8 - 10 medium-s. beets
1 cup shredded cabbage
2 large onions -
3 large potatoes -
6 tomatoes (or tom. purée)
1 Tab. sp. vinegar
1 Tbs. sugar
1 clove garlic
½ cup cooked navy beans -
1 Tbs. Flour - 1 Tbs butter -
Boil soup meats + greens in a
large pot with Water - 1 - 2 hours

Borscht recipe in Maria's writing.

Seperately cook the beats - unpealed.
then peal + cut in smal pieces.
strain the meats + cut in smal
pieces. pour the soup back in pot
add beets, cabbage and everything
els - + cook for one hour.
siken the soup with flour +
butter - serve with the bowl
of sour cream on the side.

Quick Borsch

2 cans consomme   ½ tbs worcester sauc.
1 can bouillon - ½ cup juice
1 cup water   canned beets,
1 tbs. vinegar -   ½ cup s.cream.
    bring consome + water to boil.
add vinegar, worcesta sauce, beet juice
reheat but do not boil - add
sour cream,

Quick Borscht recipe in Maria's writing.

Walking into the Happe house was an interesting and educational experience along with doing homecare.

On the walls were pictures of the Dehn home and family circa 1915-1917 in Russia. I particularly liked the picture of Lili Dehn, Maria Happe's mother, dressed in an aristocratic long dress with a train probably typical of the court of Czar Nicolas and Empress Alexandra. The women in the group pictures wore long dresses and large hats.

Each time I came I found Maria Happe peering at me as she was cuddled beneath her white down comforter.

Taking care of her was a smooth flow of personal cares.

While caring for her, she told me of her mother in the court of the Empress, her escape from the royal court to London. Her mother had a son so she was not killed by the but allowed to escape with her husband,

Letter from an aide (caregiver).

an officer of the Czar's
in London Maria was born.
She lived there until the family
had to flee this time to Venezuela.
Growing to adulthood, she became
an interpreter fluent in seven
languages. Her husband came to
Venezuela as an engineer from the
US government and Maria was
assigned to him as an interpreter.
A romance blossomed between
them and they married.
Maria and her husband lived
in Rome afterwards. She
liked it there.
When I came the first thing I
did was plug in the coffee pot
On a Christmas a we sat down
and enjoyed coffee and buchte a
jelly. All types of coffee bread
buchteln is a family favorite
of mine.
Maria was fluent in seven
languages she said for mental gymnastics
she would take a word and go
thru the same word in all
seven languages. She HAD a
memory!

Letter from an aide (caregiver).

– 2 –

In one of our conversations, we got on the topic of 4711, the cologne popular in Cologne, Germany. I told her I had been to Cologne and got a bottle which I liked. When I retired she gave me a bottle which sits on my dresser. It reminds me of her, the cares and the pleasant conversation.

Alice Svec (Svec)
BS, NA.

I had journalism in high school and creative writing in college. I was a B+ student so my writing is not probably as good as yours. I have not had any experience in writing memories. I have a pleasant memory of Maria and her family.

I hope I have the facts straight and clear as she told me.

Letter from an aide (caregiver).

Sestina by Lili Gundersen

Setting light illuminates her fading face
When we meet for her four o'clock tea.
The water boils in the other room.
She always asks for black tea,
Like Earl Grey
With a spot of milk, she sips through a straw.
Up to her dry lips the sweet drink travels.

We talk about Venezuela, Russia and the days of her travels,
Before I was born, before the wise lines of her face.
She doesn't like my darker hair. She thinks it should be blond like straw.
Her disapproval hurts me so I focus on my tea,
And I try to fill my mind with happier thoughts but there's no room.

Silence slips inside and stalks the room,
Natural at first but oh how it travels,
It clears time to study her crumpled hands and tired gray hair.
She drops her eyes from my face.
The cup falls from her grasp and spills the tea.
I sadly pick up her straw.

On the wall hangs a hat made of straw.
She wore it back when she and my grandfather still shared the same room.
Back when he was alive to accompany her afternoon tea.
She gets quiet and I see her mind travel,
To the painting above the table, to my grandfathers face.
The oil paint, under layers of dust, is beginning to look gray.

Outside the sun's departure leaves the sky gray.
My grandmother's eyes fall to her red straw.
I wish it were easier to tell her all these things to her face.
Like how I miss her old house and the yellow room
My mother used to sleep in, with shelves of treasures from her travels,
Or how I miss the time when she was the one making the tea.

I was not with her and her last cup of tea.
I think it was probably Earl Grey.
I never asked enough questions about her travels.
I think in heaven she will be able to use her hands, not a straw.
My world grew smaller. There's alot of empty room.
She was graceful as ever; there was nothing left to face.

Full of tea and travels and straw hair that turned gray,
To face a room that is emptying of her being,
Traveling to one last place.

Thoughts on Care-giving For One's Parents After Kurt's Passing

$\mathcal{B}$y being with them we resolve many things—Their heritage and our own. It is our raw material. I see them with a different perspective: Maria seems very frail and holy, and I know see that Kurt was her guardian. With him gone, I will try to be her protector but also I will see a new resilience in her, a new way of being. She is shadowed by no one and can come into her own.

It is our duty to take a contemplative and sacred perspective in caring for them. In our mid-life we have begun to experience some of the many losses in life, and in looking back and taking a tally, licking our wounds we can find our own; we take on a new non-linear way of thinking as we begin to piece together that tapestry of their lives, the essences of their beings. We internalize them and make their essences part of our own, and after all that has past with him, my father, I will be left with a lightness of being, more clarity and order; a clean space.

My father is no longer only an elder in my mind. He comes back to me in many forms: a semi-orphaned boy in pre-war Germany, a playful, fun-loving father, an international businessman returning from long journeys to exotic places with gifts for all. We must be there to hear the transmission of their stories. We must give this step validity and time. It is very essential that we receive their stories and it is time to be present for their process.

My father's Alzheimer's state did not allow for a clear transmission at the end but we did have the strong present together; the strength of the 'present moment,' as we sat side by side, became so important—a way of imprinting his stamp on myself.

If it is too difficult to be with them, if our wounds are too deep, just shorter, limited encounters can work. Visit them without our armor and preconceived notions or masks to fill curious space between us. I used all the yogic breathing that I learned, to tolerate difficult moments, and the varied range of feelings one experiences in hearing our loved one's messages.

It is important here to realize that all difficult situations are passing, but we need to meet in the moment, especially with someone who has memory loss. This is the time to say 'Bon Voyage,' and to make sure that we send them off well. Help them, your elders to complete their process so that their work does not have to pass on to our children.

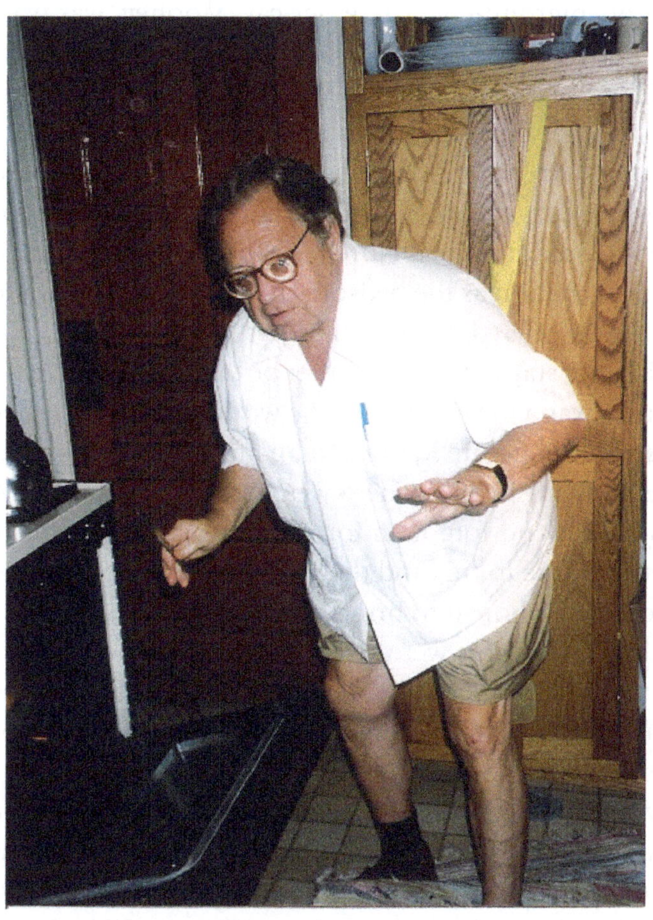

Kurt cooking, as I like to remember him

Days With Maria

$\mathcal{A}$lthough Maria revived at the center after accepting Kurt's passing, we both knew she would thrive better in her home's cozy environment. There her cat, Mooney, was waiting. Her treasures, like her Russian egg collection (marble eggs from all over the world, and a special amber one), letters from the Empress Alexandra to her mother Lili, and a Russian icon given to Lili at the time of the Bolshevik Revolution, were carefully placed along with many family photos in a prayer corner that Maria had created. She even had a small green parakeet named Fiorella that she missed there. I thought to myself that as soon as the bedsores healed with the advanced treatment the center offered, I would take her home.

During her stay at the care center both of her roommates passed away. Marion was a local artist, whose work I had previously admired and whose poised nature Maria had an affinity for. Losing these two ladies was difficult for her. There was the incident where Maria was left on the toilet and forgotten for over half an hour, which I found very upsetting. Due to this and the gloom of death, which resided on her medical hall, I hoped to bring her home.

The logistics of this were very difficult. The social work staff did not want to let her go. Finally, after repeated care conferences and her wound care sessions improving her condition, the passing of her two newly befriended roommates, and the long dark winter, we both knew it was essential to bring Maria back to her 21st street bungalow. Her estate had almost been depleted at this point due to the $8,000 or so per month it had cost to keep her at the center, so it was time to formulate the plan to bring her home. Who would be her caregivers

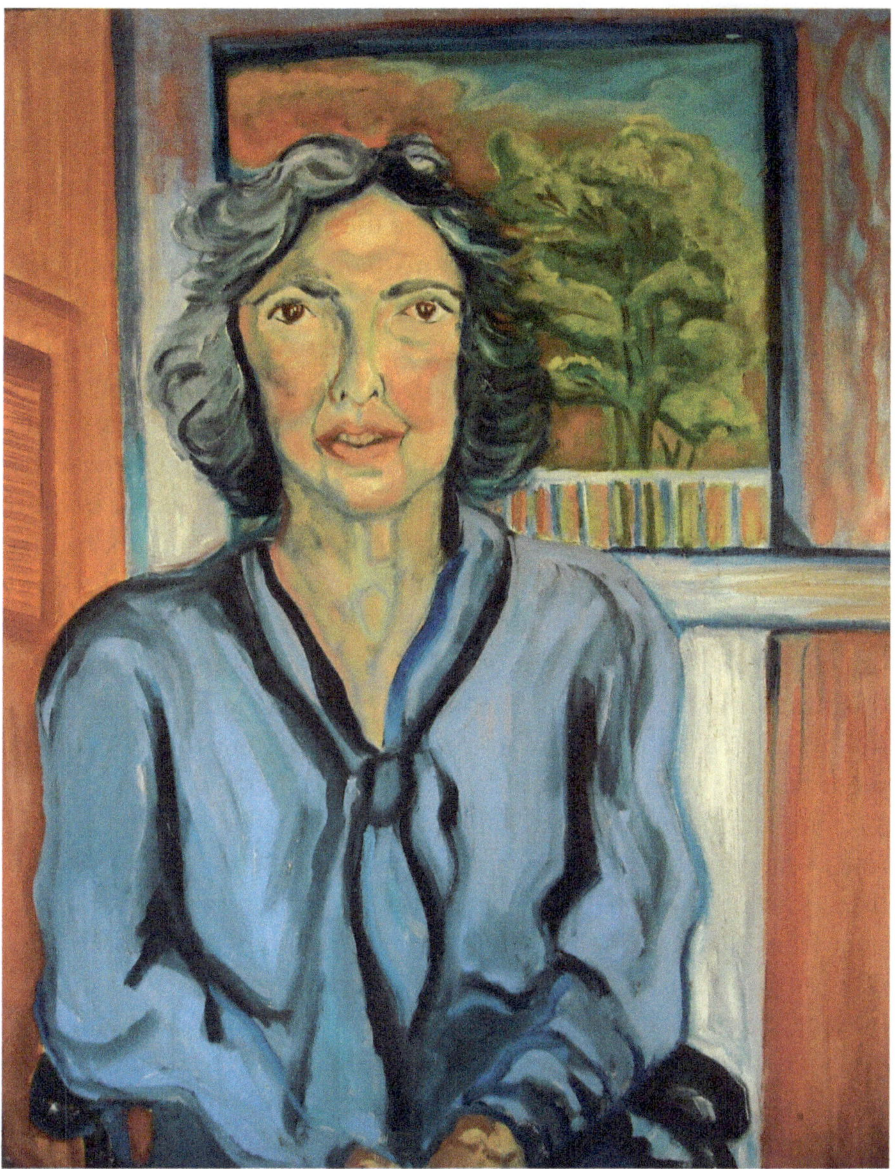

Painting of Maria by Joanie.

there? Most had moved on to other positions due to burnout after Kurt's demands and the difficulty of caring for Maria's bedsores. Although, we assumed Kurt was in a better place, and her sores had now improved, it pushed us in a new direction towards home.

As a long shot we placed an ad in the local newspaper for a helper that could provide for Maria's care at night and be a stable force in the home, for her in exchange for room and board. By taking this path we would ensure her safety and we could find a hired/or community CNA type to do the daily routine of propping her up in the mornings and using the Hoyer lift to get her going into her electric wheelchair, where she could be free to move about the house, porch, deck and garden. This would be the scope of her world.

Our ad was only answered by one man, Dan, a 30ish year old fellow who won us over at first glance. He resembled my brother-in-law so our level of familiarity with him seemed instant. However, we did not know he had a dark history of neglected child support payments to a child he fathered in his earlier years of manhood. This would eventually conflict with his ability to care for Maria. Yet, Dan was the main reason Maria could live on in her home. He was at her beckon call when he was home and in the evenings he would check on her and reposition her in her bed. The bedsores were very painful, and even with the inflated air mattress cushioning her frail body, they continued to plague her in her hip and buttock area, cause by long days of sitting in her wheelchair. Maria slept with an elaborate set up on pillows and rolls to cushion her body and Dan knew the exact placement of these and had the tenderness to move her.

We supplemented Dan's night duty with a Colombian couple from our church, Juan and his beloved wife Berta. Maria took to them instantly with her fluent Spanish. Berta, a retired scholar and poet from Bogota, often wrote and read her poetry for Maria. This relationship reminded Maria of her Caracas years and she thrived under the couples care. Berta's husband Juan was a debonair and savvy Columbian fellow with a mysterious past. He would always say, "How arrrrrre you?" with his deep Colombian accent. Maria enjoyed their company and the drama they brought to her life. Often they would all be together in the kitchen, preparing Southern American specialties, such as "Sopa de Golindrina" and other exotic dishes. (See recipe section).

Juan was able to use his Colombian work background in agriculture and livestock to work at a university run swinery, where he helped to inseminate pigs. It was rudimentary and base work. A pig attacked him as it charged him in anger; he also developed sore arthritic hands from the work. Maria would help him with special teas and remedies. The one that worked best was chamomile used in her treatment of Kurt and his evening nervousness and insomnia.

Juan was a charming South American male and we allowed him to woo us all with his lovely singing and his own poetry. I think we were all desperate for the attention at the time. Occasionally he would ask for a car ride around the neighborhood where he could romance us in his endearing Latin way. His downfall was his bipolar personality, which really should have been managed by medicine. It seems he refused to take it and this lead to some altercations with the local police. He was combative with them on occasion and even had a chase scene or two. Finally, this behavior, mixed with alcohol, led to the loss of his job in town. He found other work on a farm in the midwest later, but ended up in prison for a few months due to an overly friendly innuendo with a minor female, where he simply asked her some personal questions. In jail he was able to catch up with his readings and write many thoughtful letters; here is one of them:

Dear Joanie,

Thank you so much for your card and gift; God bless you for it…I know that you must be sad about the loss of your beloved father, but life has to go on and we must endure all the mishaps that we encounter through our journey. "Life is a journey, not a destination." We haven't been trained to deal with death as a natural process after birth. Life is not the opposite of death; birth and death are stages or turning points in life, which never ends! Never! That is the real mystery. We are tied to the process of birth and death again and again for a reason. Reincarnation may be a true aspect of life. The reason after this process is to learn and live the fact that we are one and that God loves us and that is the way it is! Once the soul learns this truth they no longer need to be born again into this material world, so it stays in a different sphere or world and becomes a co-worker with God to help others find the path to his His Infinite Love! I truly believe it is just as simple as that. Our bodies are just "borrowed" organisms or instruments to survive on earth. But Soul can endure even though the body ceases to be. That is part of our "evolution" back to the source, which is the "Ocean of Love and Mercy" which we call God. Religion means "re ligare" or "trying back to our real home which is "heaven'; this seems fantasy but it is the only truth there is!

Regarding my "crime, it was not "flirting" as you said, 'under the influence". All it is is a terrible lie from a woman who is disturbed (the girl's grandmother). The Police took her word and that is why I am imprisoned. There was an encounter with a 12-year-old girl; this is true….but not as they put it. I had not intent of having physical contact with her at all. They do not understand. They have twisted my words. That is totally false. The door was never locked! It had to be closed or else the cat would have gone out! This is just an absurd situation that needs to be cleared out and I know I am innocent! Only God knows that I am really concerned about the girl's future, because she does not have a Dad and the grandmother who is her guardian is somehow a "disturbed" person that is having all kinds of problems with the people around her. I'm not the only person she is against as she has had trouble with other neighbors. We will see how this is all cleared! Thanks again for writing, see you soon! Love, Juan

During this drama, I spend hours in the bath-tub talking on the phone, trying to calm Berta, speak to the hysterical grandmother, and Juan's lawyer…trying to justify his behavior as innocent and just one that is culturally misunderstood of a Latin American Romeo. Juan really was a stellar person. At least it is a diversion from all the other commotion in my life at that time! (Baths were my refuge then).

Berta used to get very frustrated and disillusioned with Juan's mood changes… and I would find her deeply sighing in the kitchen and repeating again and again…. Aye Juan!!!

I am mostly fond of Juan and Berta because they were very loyal to Maria and particularly in her final days.

Maria's nap time was often intruded upon by me. When I would find her resting there in the large four poster bed, with the fleece cover of pink roses and the white cat nestled next to her, I allowed my exhaustion to envelop me. I would often then nap right next to her in my father's old spot. I would find peace there, like a young child aside a loving mother. Without Kurt here, our past protector; my mother and I are bound together in a solidified force. We are surrounded by afternoon sun and dappled light in Maria's cozy room and we are assured that Kurt has arrived to his light spot above. Without speaking, to one another, we both know this.

12

As I mentioned, Berta was a poet in her own right. Here is one of the poems she wrote us:

Mother:

I know
you won't leave me in winter
because all the roads are closed,
even those in Heaven.
You will not leave me in spring;
she waits for you
with multiple colors and magical beauty.
I know
you will not leave in Summer,
you are embraced and captivated
by his warm nights and ardent days.
In Fall you won't leave,
he told me that
you will go by his arm
picking up the leaves.
Mother:
I bind you to my heart,
I withhold you.
To go away from me
you'll have to invent a new season,
a new dawn, and a new day.

Madre:

Sé que no te irás de mi lado
en el invierno porque están
todos los caminos cerrados,
aún los del Cielo.
No te irás en primavera,
ella te espera
con multiples colores
y mágica belleza.
Sé que no te irás en verano,
te enlanzan y cautivan
sus ardientes días
y sus cálidas noches.
En otoño no te irás,
él me lo dijo,
que irías de su brazo
recogiendo las hojas.
Madre:
Yo te ligo a mi corazón,
yo te retengo.
Para que tut e vayas de mi lado
tendrás que inventarte una nueva estación,
un Nuevo amanecer y un nuevo día.

BERTHA LOPEZ GIRALDO

Juan and Bertica were a godsend. They came daily to assist Maria with her tasks after Kurt had passed and she was alone— alone to become herself in her fullness. My father had dominated her the passed year, with all his needs. I had thought that he was the purpose of her living, yet he departed, she came into her own. She no longer had to be the quiet woman who lived in his shadow, but blossomed into a vibrant, capable woman. Still frozen with rheumatism, she needed companionship and help.

Juan and Bertica were sent from the local Episcopal Church, as the father there knew that Maria was fluent in Spanish and could also help them to assimilate to our culture, while they helped her with everyday tasks. It was truly a symbiotic relationship and it provided the drama that she often craved. Berta was probably older than Juan, but with all her make-up and hairdo's we dared not speculate on her age. She looked very well! She had the sense of drama expected of an artistic temperament. In Colombia, she was a published and renown poet, often submitting verses for our church newsletter. We were all part of her church Spanish class, where we put on small plays in order to practice our Spanish. Juan translated all the scripts for her. In one we recited from memory Pablo Neruda's poem "Me gusta Cuando Calles" and it became a Maria household favorite. (See page 109) as it was recited for Maria on her final day of living per her request.

Berta wrote detailed poems for all and about all of our personalities. She loved animals and eventually wrote a book on beloved house pets; dogs! At our tea parties we often recited Neruda's beautiful poem…We knew things were difficult for Juan and Bertica, in their adjusting to the U.S. culture and with their immigration papers coming through. Berta would let on with her telltale heavy sighs. When Juan left La Crosse for month-long trips to visit his daughter, She was clearly depressed. They relied strongly on one another.

The Colombian couple doted on Maria. They made her specialty foods and entertained. Maria had a lovely bird- "Fiorella," a yellow parakeet, to keep her company. I would often find them in conversation. At night, Berta would cover the birdcage with an old lace tablecloth. When we created a backyard cage and a goldfish pond to add the menagerie there, I often found the traces of them sitting on the pond's edge, feeding the fish or searching for missing fish. Juan was often in the pond in high rubber boots, rearranging rocks for landscaping.

Some of the Koi fish became rather large for their setting. In winter, we moved the fish into an indoor tank. One day, a black and white speckled Koi, who had survived 2 or 3 seasons, had become rather ill and lethargic in his movements. He was special because he always glared at us through the glass knowingly behind a spectacle-like form over his fisheye. I don't really believe in the transmigration of souls into animal forms, but it often reminded me of the way my father would try to focus on me behind his coke-bottle glasses. On the koi's sick day, I found Juan stroking the fish's side, doing some kind of fish CPR movements to revive him. Juan was truly a healer. The fish did not die!

Baba had the most beautiful deck-garden. From a few old pots and barrels, she converted the weatherworn deck into a small Garden of Eden. She filled the layer pots with cherry tomatoes and some larger ones with basil. All along the edges of the deck were rectangular pots filled with many colored inpatients, and petunias. Water filled bottles with magic grow solution filled the deck to make watering easy for Maria. One fall, when Maria seemed a bit glum, I chanced upon a clearance of colored mums at K-mart. I believe it was s blue-light special and at $1.50 a pot we soon had her deck dressed again for the autumn with about 30 mum pots....

One of our favorite pastimes was charging her battery-powered blue jazzy scooter wheel chair, and navigating the city blocks to the floral company. She would return with such fragrant herbs—marjoram, oregano, basil, thyme, and rosemary, which she used in her cooking. She insisted upon celebrating many occasions with rosemary-spiced pork or Russian borscht, or bilini filled with cheeses and caviar. (See recipes in back)

Food had always been central to my family's many celebrations and Baba never retired in this area. Although she couldn't actually complete many of the tasks the recipes called for, she would enlist the help of April or one of the other personal care helpers to create these meals. Maria suddenly became very commanding and exacting in her small kitchen. She had a way of cornering the aide (and sometimes me) with her wheel chair and insisting it be made exactly to her rigid specifications. This must have carried over from the days with my father who was our family's chef. Her arthritis had begun in those years and her gnarled hands made her clumsy. Instead she would sit very straight, always in a kitchen chair, and clearly tell my father, apron-clad and all, what spices and how much to add to his well loved old-world soups and stews.

Holidays at 330 South 21st. Street were always a big production, and with spring arrival, especially Easter, my mother's most beloved. Her sou chef was usually April, and they spent days creating the rum-raisin filled Russian-style pashka (see recipe section.) I never liked it as a child as it was so rich in cheese and rum flavors, but after I saw all of the fuss that went into it, in my later years with her it came to be symbolic of Maria, her heritage and her buoyant spirit.

My job was always to scout the area for the best cheesecloth to use for the weeping of the cottage cheese and cream cheese blend. Baba also made unique Easter bread in old cutout coffee cans, which included saffron and old raisins. It often did not rise enough, and I am sure it is because she was unable to knead it well, yet she always provided food for all of us, somehow.

Before I had my own children, I asked my mother for her wisdom in child rearing. Her response seemed very Anglo to me.

"They are very uncivilized. Children are like wild animals."

I had never reared human beings before with this superior air, but this was her stance on many things. My mother was very proper in all areas of her life. After her estate up-bringing with French tutors and then her European boarding schools; her manner was very foreign to our American culture in our rural pocket of Wisconsin. I always wondered how she fared with her proper stance.

On one occasion, I found my mother on a return from a recent clinic visit and mini-bus ride with some cowboy-of-a-driver. She was dressed elegantly in a pink chiffon blouse and pearls—once looking lovely, I am sure. Now she was covered in bloodstains on the front of her shirt.

"What happened Mother?" I inquired.

"I've had a bit of an accident en route. The minibus went over a few bumps and spilled me over in the back. I guess the driver did not tie me down."

I cringed at her disheveled appearance and her shaken stance. You can be sure I called the company with complaints and once again thought of getting my own minivan converted into a wheelchair accessible van, but without the backseat. Where would the 3 kids and dogs go?

Although Dan was the reason Maria could live on in the house, he was at her beckon call when he was home in the evenings and checked on her to reposition her body in bed. The bedsores were very painful and even with the inflated air mattress cushioning her frail body, the sores continued to plague her on her hip and buttock area. The long days of sitting in her wheelchair created these.

Maria slept with an elaborate setup of pillows and rolls to cushion her body and Dan knew the exact placement of these and had the tenderness to move her. Dan considered himself a healer and whether he really was or not, Maria believed him to be one. Mr. Dan Granger of Puerto Rican descent, with all of his strange quirks was irreplaceable. He was the reason she could remain in her home, instead of a care center. That was the choice we had made. Unfortunately, Dan came with a slew of back child support payments. His child's other refused to invite Dan into their life, partially due to the situation that he was not a good provider. Dan had a spotty history holding down jobs. I recall he did work for a canoe-making business once, but soon got into a tiff with the master builder over Dan's views on the world, or his insistent need to cure an ailment using some outlandish modality. He tried magnets, infrared, vitamin and algae supplements, and chi machines on my mother and whoever else would succumb to being his guinea pig. He could have been a full-fledged homeopath if his patients could stand his in-depth rationale for trying his suggested treatment modalities. Many times I just wanted to visit my mother, but Dan's interference regarding a new health device or gimmick was the necessary ticket in order to get to see my mother.

The one treatment I did succumb to was Dan's chi machine. It did wonders distressing and balancing my energies. As I lay flat on the old red shag carpet of the guest room floor with my ankles placed into the oscillating machine, the rotating, jiggling contraption cleared me, or at least lulled me into a soother state of well-being.

Dan's downstairs basement room was filled with a zillion diet supplements, vitamins, and powders, along with all of his magnets, and healing gadgets, and mounds of musty laundry. It was difficult to find anything or even get through the space. Occasionally, we hinted to tidy the area because the other caregivers needed to pass through there to get to the laundry area to wash Maria's clothes and sheets, but the untidiness never improved. We all managed to live with that, for we were not the one's sleeping down there. What was the most unacceptable was when Dan cornered a helper in the basement dwelling with his long-winded description of a new health remedy. He was strongly built, in a more robust way; and he may have intimidated some of the more petite helpers. One time, Dan physically approached someone from behind, while she was doing laundry and in a playful way embraced her in a peek-a-boo fashion to make his presence known. This did not go over very well with the younger gal, and she soon stopped coming to care for Maria.

One day I received a call from Maria that two police officers barged into Maria's house around teatime and inquired about Mr. Dan Granger. He was apprehended in his basement room for delinquent child support payments and a sort of paddy wagon situation. Dan was a convicted felon- five hours north in a place called Shell Lake. This was an area he once resided in and where he most likely lived with his early "family," his child and his child's mother. Dan was now placed behind bars, and Maria was living at home alone, without her mainstay helper, Dan. This was all very stressful. I am plagued with being Dan's keeper. I received a message from Dan's lawyer, Mr. Collins:

"Hello Mrs. Gundersen....Martin Collin's here. I got your card the other day, and am responding to that. I don't know what to tell you. I think the judge made it very clear that he wants you to bring Dan to court and he expects you to drive him up here to Shell Lake...and if Dan does not show up in court he may charge you with the expenses to bring him up. Theoretically, Could you be required to pay the bail of $25,000 cash if Dan breaks his bail?... I guess you can, but I have never seen that in 10 years that I have practiced law.... Why shouldn't you pay to get Dan up here? That's really what you're on the hook for. I honestly believe that Dan's ride is the issue...but if you have a problem with that when Dan goes to court next time, he could simply stay up here...and take your signature off. It has never been my attempt to mislead you. I represent Dan and not you. Realistically, I think that the most you are in for is if Dan runs or something.... having to pay the money to bring him back...you know, if you have any questions you can call me but that's the way it is...."

Although, I was prepared once more to be the substitute p.m. caregiver, or to find another one through the agency, Maria was strangely adamant that only Dan's abilities would suffice. She insisted that without him, she was done with her home stay, and a care center was her only alternative. I was surprised to hear of her stubborn stance on this, and her sheer dependence on Dan; only then did I come to realize that Dan was a sort of 'miracle' worker. At Shell Lake, we were asked to pay his bail. With the prodding of my mother, I agreed to sign the $25,000 signature bond; meaning if he escaped the state, I was obliged to cover the cost of his delinquent child support payments. I was extremely hesitant about signing and knew that my husband would disown me had he caught wind of the fact, but my supportive mother-in-law, Betty, looked at me at the moment of truth and said, "Of course, sign, You heard what Maria said, she cannot manage without Dan."

Although, we secured Dan back at home with Maria by signing my life away—I realized that if Dan escaped to Puerto Rico (his roots), or any other place, I would be straddled with payments of the $25,000 signature bond. I made him promise he would never leave Maria's side on the five-hour drive from Shell Lake. During the scenic route home to La Crosse, (scenic because I hate driving on freeways, especially in unknown territory), Dan made sure to share the latest technology in healing gadgets—magnets, infrared, chelation etc…I was glad Maria would be a recipient of all these treatments, but what she really needed to heal, was a miracle.

I am physically drained after the Shell Lake ordeal and the cloud of the $25,000 signed bond over my head. As I regain my clarity sitting by the serene koi pond in Baba's backyard, I feel the acceptance of things as they are seeping in, a kind of resolve to let it all be, as it is. I wonder who will be sleeping at Baba's tonight as a caregiver? Is Dan back on the schedule? Did Juan get another parking ticket, really? Christian, my son, wants his allowance. I see Aksel, my middle son whizzing by in the red Mini Cooper with the Union Jack flag on it. There are other things to tend to now.

A big concern is my Alopecia. What a shock it is to lose one's mane.

What color is what is left of my hair? Who knows? It all falls away. Our essence is gone then. But we are not our hair! All we have is our essence here and now, by the beautiful pond. I doze in and out of reality.

I'm thinking again that Dan's three nights in jail were not the end of the world, and maybe had some benefit. Maybe it will reform his deviant ways to society, maybe not. I did what I could to bail him out, literally. Now I am relieved. I fade off to a sweet nap by the pond.

Once Dan was reinstituted in her house, what followed were days of tea partiers and dinner buffets on Maria's porch with the grandkids and visitors from her past who had to make the last trek to La Crosse to be with her. The visitors came from both coasts and beyond. Tom, from the early days of Venezuela, Marc, from out East, who was fond of Maria's ability to endure, and of her as a mother figure. Her niece Mary came from Germany for ten days. I was impressed with her strong resemblance to my mother. Her old friend Vera came from San Francisco and said that the reason Maria got all of her health concerns is that she put everyone else first. Maybe this was true, but maybe not, for it did give back to her the loving support she needed in the later years. I believe her health issues stemmed from the stress of escaping through the iron curtain in WWII. (See Maria's war story, page 122).

*** 13 ***

*O*ne day, while I was having a catnap with Maria, the local social worker on Maria's case dropped in. I was clutching Moony, the white cat, with fear in the back room, when I heard the social worker threaten to cut services of this and that didn't happen in the house. She had the power to deem the household 'unsafe' altogether, so we lived in a kind of dread. If she had only known I was napping in the back, listening to these threats, maybe her tone would have softened.

What I found most difficult was the social worker telling us that in order to receive further county staffing support we had to "deplete Maria's estate." I found this concept difficult to trust, to spend all of her carefully preserved nest egg in order to carry on as it was. I finally hired a lawyer, Mr. Homer for a second opinion on the strategy. He did give us his blessing and reassurance that this was the system that would carry Maria till the end. We ended up getting Maria a brand new refrigerator, and some sundries in the spending down process.

July 12, '06

After removing all of Maria's helpers: Laura, April, and Rebecca, Pisces, the care agency, calls to tell me that they have been told from above to discharge helpers, that there is a "hostile environment" in my mother's home. When I hear this news, I instantly wilt. They say that Carole was attacked by April and that Bonnie was doing her job, and in the laundry room she saw Dan nude. Dan is rough with Maria, according to the social worker, and did not do as the aide

82

advised with Maria's sores. Apparently, Dan's recurrent excessive friendliness in the basement laundry room has upset some of the elderly helpers. They find his lunging out of the dark cavernous space (in only a bath towel), very disturbing. I don't blame them for feeling uncomfortable, but I also know Dan, and this is simply his way of greeting them, he is certainly overly friendly and this Labrador behavior is being misinterpreted.

With Dan picking up the agency's slack, "don't you think he is burned out?" April was in the house (I was out of town so Maria asked her to do her bills.) "What about stolen stuff?" I say there is not much to steal, all my desperate defense to protect Maria's abode.

How will we manage without Pisces Agency who staffs Maria's house with 2/3 of her scheduled aides gone? I decide to step back from the situation and recall the saying, "There is nothing that a hot bath, and strong drink, and Book of Common Prayer can't heal."

I decide to put Dan on probation with his strange behaviors and call another agency to fill in the gaps for a bit.

I pray tomorrow goes smoothly. I have been ordered to get all helpers out—'it is a hostile environment.'

"What if I am the heavy, and manage things better?" I bargain.

"No, Joan, our helpers refuse to go in there," Dixie retorts. She is the staffing head at the care agency.

Laura and Jane will still come privately, but Jane is unhappy with things… Rebecca, Dan, etc. I have 40 hours a week to staff. Sounds like Bonnie and Carole did not assimilate. (There are constant caregiver issues).

My husband's anger spills over onto me, as he sees me overly wrapped up in my mother's care, neglecting things at home. His agitation is obvious, as he can't sit still on Maria's sofa. She believes it is due to the extra cortisone/steroid cursing through his body from the bee stings he recently got (six-eight stings.) Maria tells me that all that matters is keeping our family together. She also tells me she had to cut people out of her life for certain reasons. I will remember this! I knew Lincoln had been more than supportive. He was wearing thin now.

Today, I give Baba lunch and meet one of her new helpers from Comfy Care, Julie. She strikes me as a good match for Dan.

There are so many new helpers there lately, that it is hard to keep up with things. There is only one cure all in any situation: Maria's Borscht soup!

Borscht making is on the agenda today. This is how Baba tests the stamina of her new aides. Are they good sous chefs? In the kitchen, Baba is the master chef as she directs them in the borscht making procedure, the Russian peasant way. Here is her borscht recipe, Maria's style:

- Place fat into a cooking pot and simmer
- Add one diced onion
- Dice up 8 very deep red medium sized beets
- Add 4-5 Roma tomatoes (1 can is ok)
- Dice 1 medium cabbage and add ½ to the soup
- Add enough water to cover all of the vegetables in the pot
- Add 1 T salt
- 2-3 cloves garlic (minced)
- 2 tsp majoram
- laurel leaves
- Cover the soup with a lid, bring to a boil and then let simmer for 45 minutes
- Add 1-2 meat hunks and simmer for another 1.5 hours
- Serve with a dollop of sour cream and fresh dill.

*See other favorite recipes on the Happe household in the back recipe section.

14

*D*r. Hao reminds me to make sure I have my own alone time, to cultivate my own separate life and interests away from family demands. There is a voice inside me telling me to paint more and not to be tied to care-giving demands all the time. I do admit I get satisfaction from feeding Maria with the goal of trying to fatten her up. Carrot cake with cream cheese icing is one of our favorites. Yum.

Recently, she has been complaining that the food is either too hot or too cold. Her tongue looked very shriveled; this shocks me.

Another favorite that she gave me as a child is mashed banana with lemon. Baba shares with me that her aides don't call her much when they are not on the payroll, or bother to visit. Both of us realize that they have become our social life, but may not be real friends.

I never know what the day will bring. Baba calls from her bed. She is stranded there since Dan left for work at the canoe factory, and locked the house as he left. None of the aides can get in so she is left on her own. Someone has to break-in because no one has the key to the inner porch door. I maneuver a bedroom window that is jammed one quarter of the way up in order to get in. Yet, I am too big. I feel pressure to get in to assist her with her morning needs since it is already 11:00 a.m. She at least needs her morning coffee and pills. I think of the funny saying, "That's like a rabbit trying to fit in a snake hole with a coyote on his tail." The coyote is the urgency I feel to get in there. She always sleeps next to a night table with a back scratcher, a sliced orange to chew, and water within reach for emergencies.

I dream of my mother leaning against a bay window at our old home in Washington D.C. It is a window the size of one wall, and is symbolic of her being here. She has only a thin windowpane wall between here and now and the other side. She is only waiting to be unleashed.

Dan is off for the day so I have the opportunity to have tea alone with my mother. Dan has all her fine-tuning down but I am more clumsy.

"No milk, just a bit of honey in my tea." It is always either too hot or too cold.

She is very particular about her tea service. Sometimes we even serve it in her old world fine silver set, which we all spend time polishing for her until it gleams. I am sad with our modern society; all these nuances are slipping away.

Maria takes the time to share with me about the old family estate Holowiesk in Bialestok, Poland, (Holowiesk, the old family home, page 58), a Russian orthodox church with a blue dome, a winding river and 500 year old trees encompassing a park around an old wooden home. I learned later that Bialestok was not far from "The Forest," Bialelika, which was the Tsar's hunting ground and the home of ancient trees.

Lately, Maria is dozing in and out. She had a crusty blackish-brown substance dripping down her face, which terrified me. I was sure it was old blood, but I was relieved that it was chocolate.

"Give me a piece of choc," I say, our code word for our favorite pick me up. She laughs when I tell her about the blood, and tells me I am like a child sometimes, and that I will always be her child; yet, I will try to grow-up a bit more since it is inevitable that our relation will come to an end, on this plane.

Our Estonian cousin will make the long journey to see Maria one more time. Suddenly, I must amp up the routine due to "preparing for guests." I find myself in a whirl of cleaning the pond, making soup, taking out diaper pails, making tea, dialing helpers, practicing German to speak with the guests, cleaning cat litter, petting lonely cats, losing and finding my beloved dachshund who escaped out the back alley, making mom a frittata for lunch, and praying then to God, not to give me more than I can handle.

"Don't forget to get some beer for Juan!" To top it off, Lili, my daughter calls crying to tell me how terrible she feels since her other grandmother, Betty, tells her that everyone is dying.

Often, I feel the triangle wedging me in again. For one, I feel the need to sneak over to check on Maria, either before dinner or right after, under the pretense of going to Kwik Trip or getting gas. I plan on just stopping for a moment, but there is always something zany going on in my mother's house. The hearing-aide on the nightstand is beeping, calling for new batteries, or the new helper will only make the eggs, but feels uncomfortable feeding them to Maria. So on my quick check in, I tidy a messy room, or feed Maria something, and put in a load of laundry. Once I found Berta passed out on the sofa and Maria was consoling her.

I have a dream where a voice tells me to "turn down the static." There is too much noise in my world and I hope for just a bit more peace. There is a voice inside yelling at me to go to my studio to make art…and to check in with the rambunctious teens at home more. Soon there will be a clearing in the clouds above, and I will find more time for all this. I see that my elder's dimming is telling me to shine stronger. Our light in unison must not fade, however.

Our Uncle Michael visits. He is Maria's nephew that grew up in Argentina after being displaced from Europe after WW2. He enlivens her household by giving all of us tango lessons on her living room floor. We clear out furniture so that the living area and dining room becomes a dance floor. She is the audience that we try hard to please. We want to revive her a bit. Violeta and Francie, another friend are led across the dance floor. Violeta adds drama by adding a quick sharp tango kick before her turn. Michael has become a proficient dance teacher, and before long we are all moving across the floor to tango. Maria, once a fine dancer, comes out of her doldrums to enjoy the festivities and music.

I come to realize that it is the little things that save us each day. Today it is that my mother is smiling again and she looks well in one of her comfy pastel turtleneck sweaters, by her indoor geraniums that she babies, sitting there by the sunlit window. She is like one of the plants, taking it all in for vitality. April is in the back kitchen making us popcorn. All is well for now!

15

fter this phase of well-being, and Uncle Michael's departure, I note how skinny my mother has become. She is disappearing in front of my eyes. We all load her with ice cream, spoon-feeding her desperately, but she is unable to keep weight on. When I ask Dan what he thinks of Maria's state, he always responds with one blanket statement, "I don't know."

We have all become so intertwined day to day, that we no longer really see things and Maria as she really is. October 8th is the day her mother died, and I pray that she will linger a bit longer with us, fighting my superstitious nature.

Today when I visit, Maria has her teeth out and I see her in a true light. She is groggy today, leaning over the side of her chair. I drop off some cookies for her, but she tells me she is afraid of choking. I realize now by her tired and emaciated appearance that her days are few. I must prepare myself for when I hear, 'she's gone.' I hope it happens quietly in her sleep.

Her mouth and teeth are causing her so much discomfort. It seems like if she could just get dental treatment, maybe she could recover. Other issues are that the 'pill key' is missing. Laura sounded weird and aloof last night; maybe she knows where the key is to the green metal pain pillbox so I can get her a pain pill to relieve her pain. There is little I can do now and things seem rather dismal as she is slumped by the TV in her dark home, waiting for 8:30 or 9:00pm when a caregiver can make it to slip her into bed. My only remedy, or quick fix, is to slip her a spot of tea.

I see helpers have been resistant to taking the messy kitchen trash out. I run it out to the alley as I go, knowing when I get home there will be more trash for me to take out there, and probably a sink full of dishes and an unloaded dishwasher. "Moving mountains," is the message I would remind myself of during the feat I had to accomplish here.

16

*B*aba has a very long Christmas list this year, as she insists on buying presents for all the helpers. There must be at least 10 different ones on her list. She also insists on making the beet and herring salad. It has grown on me over the years. The infamous herring recipe can be found in the recipe index.

When I see Baba today, she is sunning herself in the Kitchen with Dan.

"Please go to the cupboard and get Dan his Christmas gift."

It is a funny little bear with cash stuffed into its vest.

"Don't forget the herring salad, and don't put orange with the cranberry sauce. It doesn't go with beef." Christmas preparations have begun. I am thrilled to have found a small symmetrical tree at Kmart for Baba's house. That will lift her spirits. She has a very long Christmas list this year as she insists on buying presents for so many helpers. We also all get together to make the Xmas Beet and Herring salad. (See recipe index for Herring Salad)

I am amazed at all of her culinary knowledge.

As I leave, Dan suggests that I order Tupperware from HSN cooking show because it is the 'day's special.' Baba is mopey because Juan has been charged with a felony for some kind of bar scene, and then fleeing from the police officers. Imagine the scene of the Colombian gaucho cowboy fleeing the law. This makes it easier to understand. With a felony charge, Juan could be out, possibly deported, or suffer a huge fine. As I walk out the door, I say "Love you" to Baba as my new good-bye words..

Baba says that her mouth is very dry, and she feels poorly. I lead her outside for some fresh air. For some reason, when we speak to one another I am unable to look directly in her sad, intelligent brown eyes. I try to, but it is difficult to do so. Is it because I can read the truth in them, and she in mine? What is too hard to share in our reality? Baba has told me to look into my loved ones eyes always, for who knows if it will be the last. Our eyes cannot lie to one another as easily as our voices can. There is so much reality to our human pain.

I must run home before Lincoln gets there from work, all tired and cranky. It makes it much worse if I am not there on his return. He accuses me of spending most of the day at my mother's place. He resents my lack of focus on our own home and family. This becomes an issue in our marriage, and I often have to lie to check on Maria. I tell him I have to run to Kwik Trip for some cream or cat liter. I hate this situation, but it is what I must do to manage everything that is on my plate. Is this what Christians call 'The Cross' we must carry?

My old Aunt Kitty, who would visit us from Caracas once told me, "If you don't do anything all day, always make up the bed." I think she thought it makes a clear statement that you value your marriage bed, and that you did do <u>some</u> housework, even if all else is in disarray, or maybe it is about beginning 'a new' everyday in your marriage or life. It's true meaning still eludes me.

As the day's helper tries to wrap up things at 330 S. 21st street to leave, Maria asks for one more thing. "Jane, Can you put a bit of honey in my tea? Just a bit."

As Jane turns back to do this, I try to lift her spirits. "Mom, your hair looks good." What is it about women, especially elder ones that are so very hair focused? I suppose I won't have this concern if my alopecia keeps me hairless. Maria then asks me to brush it, just a bit off her forehead. It had lovely silky texture, and I regret not cutting a bit off for a relic of her in case I lose her soon. It reminds me of many mornings of my girlhood where she would brush my waist long hair at the dark wooded vanity in her bedroom. She would ask my sister and I, "Do you want it back? Down? Braids-up?" Doing our hair was our before school ritual that I came to love. Just as I attempt to head home to dinner preparation for my own family,

Juan pops in after being saved for now from the felony charge by a loyal church member. He asks, "Could you do me a favor? I need a cigarette at the Kwik Trip."

"Not now Juan. I have to get dinner going, but I promise to drop them by later."

I think I have made my escape. I must look like an easy target in my not quite right wig and white snow ball-like fluffy Christmas sweater.

"What brand?" I ask.

"Newport Shorts." He yells back.

There are some uncovered mysteries still that I need to uncover with maybe not much time. It is important to ask all of the questions. I usually had one in mind before I visited.

"Mom, was childbirth terribly difficult for you?"

I know she had complicated pregnancies with her RH-factor and toxemia, and even 1-2 miscarriages. Another one was,

"Where was the most favorite place that you lived? Poland? Venezuela? Rome? D.C.? Here?"

Many of my friends had accused me of having a father in the CIA.

"Are you sure dad wasn't in the CIA, Mom?"

He was always away, traveling to some exotic locale, Beirut, Nigeria, Libya, Brazil, Ecuador, Colombia…

"No, Darling. He worked for Northrop as an engineer, I am sure."

It is feast or famine over there. Today, I find Berta, Juan, Dan, and Ophelia, the 80 year old, rotund, Mexican neighbor, with mild dementia. What lovely company for Maria today!

I have been attending more funerals lately. Maria despises them, so does not go. At an elderly family friend's service the minister who presides, told the mourners that Jesus is the host and the departed is being catapulted into space to be aside the lord. All that knew her must count their personal loses and gains at this point in time of their loved ones departure, (not only material of course.) That is the job for those left behind and also to keep her essence alive by sharing memories and speaking of them, when the opportunity arises; They clearly must not be forgotten.

17

I have a telling dream. I am struggling to get my parents into a van from the back hospital entrance. There is too much heaviness, their weight, her cumbersome electric wheelchair; the steel delivery doors are all immovable. We are waiting, including my husband- anxiously waiting for some kind of assist. Two more agile ladies go before us. I cry out for help in an exasperated tone. The driver tells me that tears won't work. I awake in a frustrated, combative mood.

The last night was very creepy and eventful. After a soccer game in the rain, receiving pink carnations from my boys, sitting with Mrs. Craemer, the mother of Christian's friend and hearing about the boys making volcanoes, Marina calls me to let me know that Jane and Dan told her that Baba has been choking on her pills. I see her end? Like this?

I wait a long moment to let reality hit, and then I drive down to her house. It's the beginning of a very long escapade. Firstly, the ambulance carts her away. I meet them at the hospital. The med-flight paramedic does a test on her to prevent any oppressive measures. I sit tightly by her like a lioness guarding her prey, or cub. The loyalty is strong. I will not leave her side. I am unbelievably there for her. I won't let any foul play or mistreatment occur. I know my medical lingo, and the doctor, Dr. Cooper, is cool and nice, and cautious with mom. There is nothing aggressive in his manner. He requests Dr. Unser like my dream, I grapple with the "no code." lot's of phlegm comes up; I dread losing her here on this bed in the E.R.

I am extremely calm. There is a full house in the room- lots of people coming and going- caregivers. I see Marian- a familiar face, it empowers me somehow. I am "in," being a physician's wife. Much sputum comes up. This is unnerving. I worry about her aspiration. I argue with Dr. Cooper about the middle road choice. We agree to do an endoscopic tracheo throat procedure. We wait for a long time.

She is skeleton and bone, falling to the side, yet dressed cheerily in a brightly colored Indian jacket. She hears mildly and has a impotent, raspy voice. I'm concerned about her having pneumonia. I sit reading "slow cooking tips." I tell her to sleep. She needs repositioning. The male nurse in the room is gruff but helpful. He helps with the green phlegm from her sinusitis, or is it bronchitis? What about the pills? (I mention aspirate, and Dr. Cooper reacts.) There is risk, and I am the power of attorney in my mother's healthcare. I'm her advocate.

This is invasive. She wants to take a sedative, and I see the scope plunging down her, a probe with a light, down a windy tube of swirly-coiled flesh. It is her tonsils. I watch the screen, and feel as if I am on a slow rollercoaster ride down a tunnel. We are traveling within Maria. I'm not sure why the doctor insists that I stay. I get a grip. Thank God for the smooth silk sheen of the magazine to tether me to the world of stability, reality, hope. "No pills seen, but maybe they were dislodged.

"Time is like rafts strung together," my Discover Magazine reports. This must mean that it is only fathomed in sections or that it is strung together by it's separate parts as a patchwork fabric of many colors.

She gasps– no sedatives; I have consented to her pain. Is there a mix of fear and remorse and pleasure in this– just a flash. The mother–daughter primal tie is what awakens the pleasure! This surprises me, but I writhe in pain with her. It is done; the pills are gone. She has survived the soothing gas, the IV's, and this odd procedure of tunneling. I thank my enthusiastic doctor and his aides. Mom–Mom–Mom!

The 6 West transport– I'm asked many questions about her lifestyle. I answer while she dozes. The Indian medical student, Dr. Marino takes a thorough and personal assessment.

"Do you have a living will? What are her desires? "

I change the topic to my dream of visiting the Taj Mahal, and I leave my mother to rest of the night. On my drive home at 2:00 am cop pulls me over. I tell him about my frail mom, and he lets me leave with only a warning. When I get home and crawl into bed, my husband's sleep–filled state is all I see. I feel my little dog, Tootsie, rolled up like a donut awaiting me, and I fall fast into a deep, healing slumber.

Baba's decline is evident after Christmas this year. She insists that I come over and show her the Norwegian bunad that I wear as a holiday costume for my husband's family Christmas party. She is very complimentary of all the embroidery and my wavy blond wig. She approves of this Scandinavian look. I leave her watching a movie with Dan. They are watching a romantic selection called "The Notebook," so I feel she is in good company.

The next day I bring her some leftover krumkakke– the Norwegian ringed tower desert. It is difficult for her to eat it due to teeth pain. She looks drawn and depleted. She tells me, "This is no way to live."

I give her bony body a hug and she seems so frail in her wheel chair. My Florida trip looms vaguely ahead. I wonder if I should leave her like this. We chitchat to blunt any discomfort. Today our conversation is about the Queen of England. My mother recalls that she was once sweet and young, but became hardened with time. She apparently related to animals better than people. She was defiantly quieter in her ways than the flashy Diana. Baba reminds me that I don't like illness or sick people. I would be a lousy nurse. It adds to my disillusionment since the dentist does not return my call. Her mouth and gums are so swollen and uncomfortable with her achy teeth that she can barely eat.

I call my sister for her support and tell her I am sending Maria to Keswick, the care center in Baltimore that she always tried to tempt us with. Keswick has Jacuzzis on each floor and Keswick has lovely views. This is only to nudge Marina into the conversation now for support…..

I run to the local Walgreens to get Maria some teeth rinse, teeth numbing solution, comfy wipes and aspirin.

The next day, Jean (Jean is April's mother and has been our devoted helper and friend) tells me that Baba told April she loves her.

April is bringing Baba a shawl, lemon and glycerin swabs. She can no longer get her teeth in, and her mouth seems glued shut.

Baba insists that I go on my mini trip even though she continues not to eat much, and has swallowing difficulty. I really needed to focus on my husband for a bit, and it had been forever since we left town together. I feed her a mashed banana, and plan to take her to the dentist on Monday when we return. It will only be 3 days and I truly believe I will see her again.

Dan is acting very nonchalant about her condition and is busy promoting pod community living to another aide. He is really ahead of his time. Dan gives me his blessing to go and leave without drama; I would not have if I didn't really believe I would see Baba again Monday.

I pray to "hold her." I do pray while I am away. I hope for sun and light to stream in to revive her, and cheer her while I am away. The sky is bleak white and heavy, laden with snow. My dear friend Mindy promises to check in or have tea with Maria. This is reassuring.

I would randomly read passages of the Bible on low days, for comfort. This one resounds strongly, and was healing– Matthew 12:

"Come to me, all that are weary and are carrying a heavy burden and I will give you rest. Take my yoke upon you and learn from me– for I am gentler and humble in love, you will find rest."

MARIA'S FAREWELL

*M*om is miserable. She is preoccupied with her own death. She is often listless, with her eyes shut, assuming a fetal position in her electric chair. Closing off, in a muffled voice, she tells me she loves me, to say goodbye.

I dance around her sad condition, make tea, tidy... It's steeped too long, or too short, I can't remember, Earl Gray or a mild herbal. She is focused on the minutiae of life; a probable distraction. The water is too hot, or not cold enough. Fat straw, thin straw– which one?

She hovers around a straw, and has hesitation over allowing food in. A pill is stuck. I feel queasy. I see her dozing with the straw in her mouth. Is this some sort of deliberate punishment on her part due to her end stage? I will not play along. I head for the bathroom for a moment of privacy, to regain composure.

This is where it gets hard.

I enjoyed the evening on my own, to regroup. I looked through old papers, the map of Holowiesk. 'How ironic,' I think, as we search for an ancient map to her roots–her childhood home, "Holowiesk."

Poor thin Mooney, the kitty, is also dissolving. She has been a good cat. Dan's trite; "I don't know," he says when questioned about the cat's status. Have all of the questions been answered? Have all of the stories been told? I wonder. Maybe it is time to call hospice, but later we decide against this as it would require a complete change of guard, all new helpers.

Tonight, when I talk to Baba I say, "Sleep well. See you in the morning."

She says, "Let's hope so."

Those tacky and rude comments verify the hostility she feels when we are not there doing things for her, and I do not step in due to needs at home (i.e. trying to have a life—whether it be nourishing friendships out of hers) Yet, it's a conundrum since she suffers from socialite jealousy I can't talk too much about away relationships—away from her. I can't really have a life, which does not include her.

"I have never been to Canada," she retorts.

No mum, but you have been many other places.

I tell my friends that she is a bit frozen in her body. It is a miracle everyday she is here but at my cost it seems. My husband reminds me of this, but it is what it is. My cross. Lincoln's father carried his grandmother into the house for dinner for two years, due to M.S. Lili is still here and we clarify some more things. She says dad and I fight less. I look forward to sweeter, deeper relations with friends. I do.

Baba is acting rather unkept and mopey, having a bowel movement due to the yogurt. She is very bowel-focused these days. I am depleted and can only visit for one hour. I feel tired. No excuses from any of the helpers to do their job. Baba has high expectations/ demands of everyone, and is burning some aides out. We all tire around her, but are enveloped by her captivating mind. Despite all her handicaps, she is very sharp.

I leave with resistance on a conference meeting with my husband for just three days, when I get a voice message from my mother-in-law.

"Your mother looks yellow today, Joan. You'd better get back here right away."

I call home to hear Maria's reassuring and selfless voice.

"Enjoy your time away darling. We can manage."

I need the rest and break, so I tell myself its o.k. to go.

I did make my mistake by leaving my mother at this precarious time in her health. She insisted I take a break and go, and maybe she did this as a window of opportunity of sorts. In prayer, I held Maria, my beloved dachshund, and Maria's helpers in a golden light. I asked that they all be sustained, while I take this time away to breathe the clear ocean air, but her will and God's will overrode.

This old Hollywood Beach Hotel, built in 1927, the same era of my mother's birth looms like a dinosaur on white, expansive Lauderdale Beach; an old lady amidst suburban sprawl. While Lincoln is at his meeting, I get a henna tattoo of a seahorse on my ankle. While Lincoln and I are finally getting to relax in the hotel's hot-tub, a fake, large-chested female in a mini golf skirt strolls by, chomping gum and flashing herself. Lincoln smiles and says "what a prize, every guy should want a big boob blonde." I say yes, but you have a false brunette also a size D, and I can easily change to a blonde, as hair is an accessory! This is one perk with having alopecia.

Later Christian, my youngest, and I take a bus. On the bus ride, Christian takes the opportunity to tell me a thing or two. He is a silent 14 year old usually, so I take the opportunity to hear him out.

"You spend too much time on the phone, micromanaging Baba and her stuff."

After shopping at the Levi Store and a dress shop, (where I am drawn to a black V cut dress) he surveys my purchases and says, "You shop too much."

Once could write a whole book on mothers and sons, that unusual dynamic. I dwell on the new black dress. Is this symbolic of what is to come very soon with my beloved mother? She always told me how difficult it was to be at her skeletal mother's bedside, and watch her pass into the next realm. She clearly stated that she did not want to do this to her own daughter—yet it did not seem right that I not be there for and with her.

The conundrum of Baba not eating irks me. I had hoped that my taking this distance on things there with her condition would bring me some clarity. The day in and day out of things made the truth of the matter illusive. It is clear to me that she must get more nutrients in her system to sustain her frail being. I was definitely emotionally drained from the daily innuendos of the situation—

"I can't swallow."

"It's too cold," or "It's too hot."

"Please heat the banana."

On our return to the old hotel, I stop in the very odd, but fascinating lobby nature store. Inside there's a taxidermied silent owl and yellow fox, and many rocks and crystals. The bearded elder hippie-type man with a kind face takes me to see the bird egg collection— a quail egg, a Kiwi bird egg, and suddenly I see it—a divine ostrich egg, perfect in form and color. For years I have wanted to possess one again, since the one my father brought from his African travels had cracked. Here she was, and my Florida mission felt complete. I had her bagged and packed, and soon she will sit on our fireplace mantel in Wisconsin.

When I call home later Aksel, who has recently visited Baba, tells me that they shared some ice cream together and she continues to feel sick. She tells him, "Life is like one long movie. It just goes on and on and on and on, and seems never to end."

This is her message to us all, that she has had enough. Her pain meds are making her very groggy. I feel the urge to hop on the first plane back, but my emotionally starved of maternal and wifely attention son and husband keep me occupied. Dan reassures me again, "She is okay."

I continue to pray and have to have her held in golden light until I return.

I feel that I am being held in some kind of cushioned world of this strong fortress by the sea, the Hollywood Hotel, as I am helpless to my mother's condition. In this pastel fortress by the sea, I come to realize that I must let Baba's illness take its course. I can't really intervene. It may be her destiny, and I must let go, yet, I don't want to, but there may be little that I can do.

It is most likely best that I am here, since I'm not sure how much help I would be. My anxiety about all this is unsettling. I meditate on the boat scene print over the hotel room's bed. All is a Caribbean blue green and pastel décor world around me. I open the window, let the sea breeze in, and fall into a needed slumber.

In the morning Lincoln heads off to his meeting, and Christian and I decide to sit by the pool. It is a cool day on the beach so I wear a sweater and leggings. I never try on my new black dress, as it seems to be symbolic of something inevitable that I don't want to face. Robin, the R.N. on the scene calls me with news that Baba continues to be very uncomfortable. She is not up for talking now. I am relieved not to be there, because I don't know how to make her more comfortable. Jane's report is that getting her up was hell, so Dan came to her assistance. I decide after watching some punk looking gulls on the beach dive bomb for food that I will leave a message on Dr. Unser's voice mail, so he can try to see if there is anything that can be done now or even first thing Monday morning.

Here is the list of my mother's symptoms:
1) Poor appetite
2) Difficulty swallowing
3) Mouth sores
4) Teeth pain
5) General achiness all over
6) Leg rash
7) Bed sores
8) No fever (Dan always said that fever was due to bowel movements)

Every time I got a call from home, I would tremble. My instinct knew it was time. I remind myself that she has worn her body out, and she would be free of suffering. I am hopeful that she will wait for me.

At 5am or so, I get an early morning call that Baba is gone. The news causes a convulsion of tears and sadness. She is gone, but along with the overwhelming sadness, I am secretly relieved. I know her body was completely worn out, and she braved her pain very strongly. She is being greeted by her mother Lili, Kurt, her brother Ali, her father-in-law Oscar, and the pets; even Mrs. Bouroff, the white Russian who became all of our surrogate grandmother in D.C. She misses and loves us all immensely, but it is time for her to fly free from her useless body now.

We both came to this world of knowing there was no way to carry on this was any further for either of us. Hardness formed between us that filled this envelope of knowing. I had others to tend to, and myself getting older and less able to withstand the tiredness, the pressures etc…the constant gnawing concern about my beloved one's well-being.

The morning of knowing she is no longer with me on this earthly plane, I find the release of tears a flood. Trying to eat the pancake and egg breakfast with the boys is impossible through the waves of grief rising. We walk back to the old hotel where I find myself at the shore with semi-warm salty waves beckoning me in. That is all I need, the salt of my tears to meld with the salty ocean water.

As I give into the gentle waves, I feel a breeze fluttering around me. The breeze, waves, mist, seem to be teasing me in, almost dancing with me, and then I hear Baba's full laughter, and I know it is she. My mom is all around me, playing with me as if I am a toy, letting me know that she is finally free of all that bound her. I feel her lightness, and joyfulness at the moment, and I suddenly find myself so exuberant with this surge of positive spiritual energy, being tossed now by an unexpected wave that swishes my boyish hairpiece in the surf and then tie a towel around my bald head—somehow cleared from the immersion in the salt and the sensation of my mother's new found liberty. All is well now, but the tears continue to flow and cleanse.

On our return home, I rush quickly to the house where I find a strange, soft candle lit room, created by helpers, Laura and April. I see her body there, made up and peaceful, with the butterfly scarf wrapped around her neck. We have had a special 2-½ years together, where we have protected one another. Before she left, Dan told me she hugged a small heart shaped cushion and spoke of abundant love. She told Aksel to live on, Berta: to be happy with things; for Dan: to find love; to April: when it is time to die, go and don't linger. She again had reiterated to her helpers that she could not handle being with her mother for her last breath, so it was better this way for her.

She had refused to talk to me when I called the last night, for it was too difficult. Berta read her poetry of choice: Pablo Neruda's 'Me Gusta Cuando Calles."(See page 109) Maria took us all under her wing and made our problems her own, and translated the solution with her worldly perspective. She was made of steel, and she tried to conceal her own suffering from us, only wanting us to see what she wanted us to see.

I do not regret not being at her side, for this was more my style. Yet, my eldest friend's mother Keke reminds me, "You were in your bed. She was in her bed asleep for the night, where you would have been in Wisconsin. One cannot know the moment of one's death."

This consoled me greatly. She left a note for us all, "no matter what happens in life, just keep moving," and she did this in her jazzy, blue electric wheelchair with the 'horse-power' bumper sticker on the back.

Baba's Passing dream

*B*aba, Anna (my niece), myself, and my sister are traveling in Machu Picchu, identifying exotic birds and plants, taking in the views, the rock formations of the Mayan ruins, and the lush abundance when Anna asks Maria a spiritual questions,

"Why must we die?"

Maria responds,

"At the end of one's journey one is often like a broken toy that no one wants to play with, and one becomes very tired. Rest is truly welcomed by the old one.

Lost in the Muddle — Joan's poem

There is not much time for talking
stories of a past
nor taping or tea
just the mess of transferring the assets,
misplacing social security numbers
clearing up bills
and finding errors and cheaters
$300 to rent the Hoyer-lift she hated using
$400 for the bed sore-cushion
That which Medicare would not pay.
You should be
Floating on air
but it is unaffordable
until you come home
if you come home
They will proclaim this
at the care conference
If you can manage
to leave the place
maybe the only out is
passing to the next space
like dad did
after only 6 weeks of
being restrained
Alarms on getting up
Swinging in mid-air
neither here nor there
As I grapple through
paper receipts
Water your flowers
Feed the cats
Try to talk to lawyers
About why the nest egg
you so tried to save

must be eaten up
appease the neighbors at
an empty home
long grass, stray cats, no night lights.

In the midst of all this
There is less and less time
For "us"
To really speak and understand
 what has and is happening
In our final time, together
Lost in the muddle
Life is strong at a point—
Vibrant, alive, active
Breathing
Then it becomes quieter
and quieter
skin is transparent and tissue thin
(there may be a slight rattle)
it leaves like the wind
thru the mouth
before than thru the ears
and maybe eyes
before it finally goes
completely

AFTERTHOUGHTS:

I have heard it said when a loved one passes you have to do the living for them, while honoring their perspective. It is important to speak about them whenever the opportunity arises; use their words and expressions (also, revive there recipes). It is healing for those left behind.

I felt an aching sense of loneliness possibly like an orphan now, realizing the umbilical cord has been cut and I am now fully grown. We are cut free now to drift, as we will. Our parents protected us and now it's our turn next. Somehow the winds seem harsher now. Even if I denied grief it would always win as it surfed through any blocks. The advice to handle this new phase was to accept the new world, but cradle yourself. By journaling in an alone space I was able to dip into the well of grief.

The moon is full and it is the dark of winter–early February. There are no signs of spring. I have faith that I will be sustained through this darkness and find my way. I continue to sense her happiness about where she is and is certain she will be recovered by heavenly hosts.

At the very end, I was told that she asked if it was snowing out, and they told her it was. She then asked for a bit of alone time before resting through her last night that last February.

After my mother's death I found my life completely changed. When she and my father moved from Bethesda, they closed our family home in the Washington suburbs to come to La Crosse, Wisconsin to be closer to their daughter (myself) and her family–It would be the beginning of a decade of intensified personal relationships that would forever transform me and the road I was on. Not only did we become interdependent again as I had as a child, but our bond was forever sealed. Through this period of time where I watched them transform from able adults to the ravages of Alzheimer's with my father and my mother's physical body giving into the ravages of a life's struggle with R.A. Although both these conditions were potentially devastating, the trials we had together in keeping things afloat were the events that empowered us throughout their final days.

I won't write this as their caregiver, but as their daughter; our roles did not really change as some say occur. They were never like my children. They were consistently to reinforce my own backbone for future reference. I saw their almost daily life for this decade and found there always an entrancing dimension to my own life. At the time I was also raising one robust family of 3 kids with my husband being an on-call physician whose life was mostly 'his work.'

"Mom, I'm here, what's happening today? Do you want me to put the water on for tea?"

"Mom" to me, but "Maria" to the cast of helpers that helped my mom get put together in his wheelchair. She had the air of a queen due to her aristocratic background from the line of General Kutuzov. Despite her chronic battle with R.A., she was always straight, poised, and well put together. She even made the Kmart sweaters that she frequently draped with a strand of pearls from Rome, look elegant.

Now that both of my parents are gone and time has passed, I know one thing that is certain– Despite the many challenges and tribulations of their last years with me, I feel their presence greatly enhanced and enriched my being and life, despite difficulties. Rumi, the poet, wrote: "Let the water settle– You will see moon and stars mirrored in your being." They are moon and stars now mirrored in my being.

After my parents passing, the world did change. I needed to go under again for some time, to honor these feelings of grief– to cradle oneself. Ophelia, at Maria's service suggested I rent her small spot in a quiet neighborhood for a bit to make a gallery/studio. The White Moth Gallery emerged, where I not only held shows and art gatherings, but also found a sanctuary to write, meditate, paint, and pray–all ways to meets the grief of this profound loss. In our final separation with our loved ones, we all leave our old world and are freed into a new path.

Pablo Neruda- Chile
Me gustas cuando callas

Me gustas cuando callas
Porque estas como ausente,
Y me oyes desde lejos, y mi voz
No te toca.
Parece que los ojos se te hubieran volado
Y parece que un beso te cerrara la boca.

Como todas las cosas estan llenas de me alma,
Emerges de las cosas llena del alma mia.
Mariposa de sueno, te pareces a mi alma,
Y te pareces a la palabra melancolia

Me gustas cuando callas y esta's como distante
Y estas como quejandote, mariposa en arrullo.
Y me oyes dede lejos, y mi voz no te alcanza.
Dejame que me calle con el silencio tuyo.

Dejame que te hable tambien con tu silencio
Claro como una lampara, simple como un anillo.
Eres como la noche, callada y constelada.
Tu silencio es de estrella, tan lejano, y sencillo.

Me gustas cuando callas, porque estas como ausente.
Distante y dolorosa como si hubieras muerto.
Una palabra entonces, una sonrisa, bastan.
Y estoy allegre, alegre de que no sea cierto.

Translation:

It pleases me when you grow silent
As though you were absent.
And you hear me from afar, and my voice
Does not touch you.
It seems that your eyes have flown from you
And it seems that a kiss has closed your mouth.

As everything is filled with my soul
You emerge from everything filled with that soul.
Dream butterfly, you resemble my soul, and you resemble the
word melancholy.

It pleases me when you grow silent and are as if far away.
As if moaning, butterfly lulled to sleep.
And you hear me from afar, and my voice does not arrive.
Let me quiet myself with your silence.

Let me speak with you also with your silence,
Clear as the lamplight, as simple as a ring.
You are like the night, quieted and clustered with stars,
Your silence is of the star, so far away and simple.

It pleases one when you grow silent, as though you were absent.
Distant and dolorous as though you were dead.
One word then, one smile is enough.
And I am happy, happy that its not so.

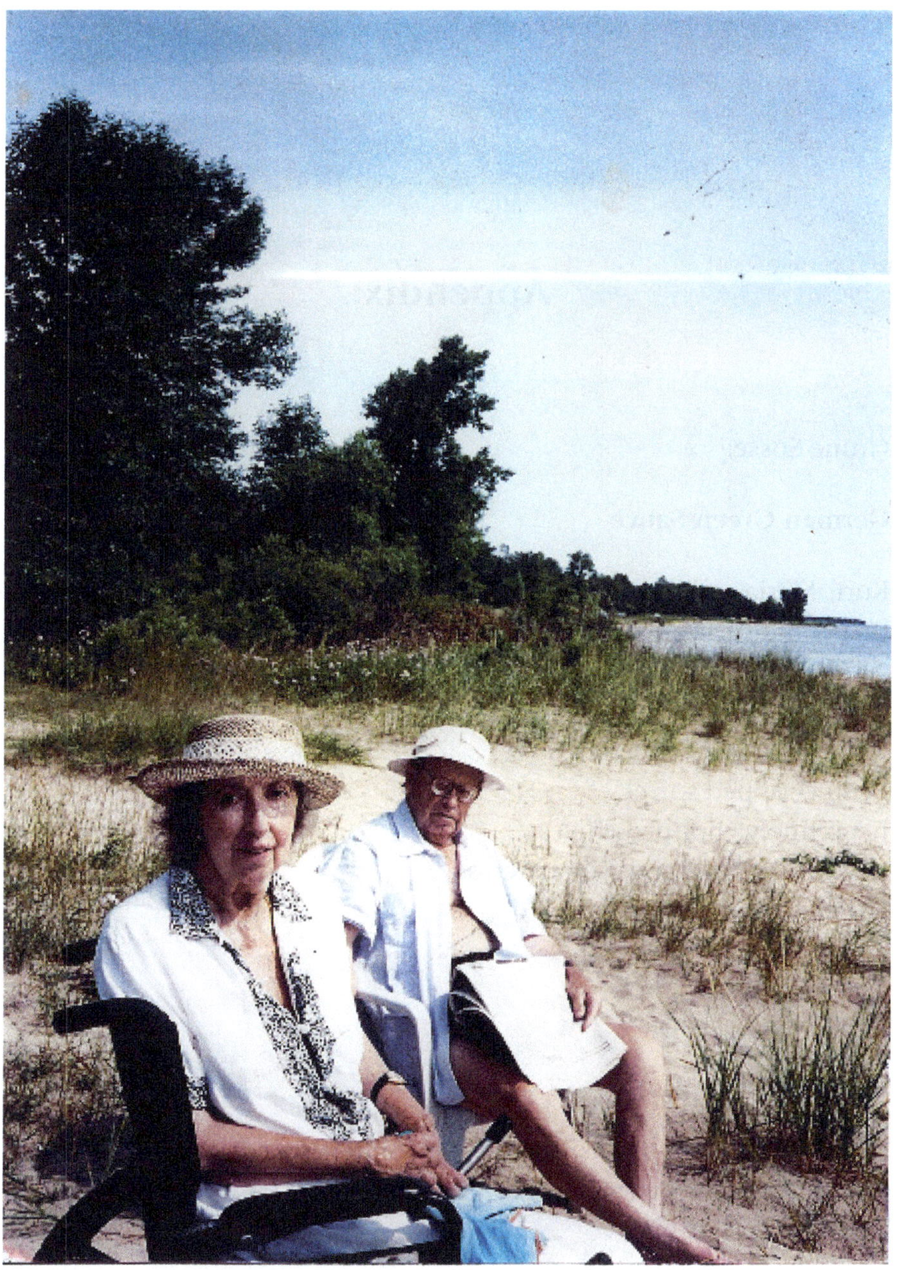

Door County shot of Kurt and Maria on the beach.
One of their favorite places to be.

Appendix:

Grune Sosse:

German Green Sauce

Kurt, Maria and Roli made this every spring with the freshest herbs that could be found. A variety of herbs can be used. Freshness is key.

2 cups parsley
1 ½ cup packed watercress
I cup chopped sorrel
I cup finely chopped chives
I handful of dill and or watercress
Celery leaves cut fine
1 clove garlic
1/3 cup plain yogurt
½ cup mayonnaise
1/3 cup milk
1 ½ tsp olive oil
1 hard-boiled egg
Salt and pepper to taste
1 clove garlic

Process green herbs and yogurt, sour cream, mayonnaise, milk egg yolk, and season with garlic, salt and pepper. Chop the hard egg whites into the sauce at the end for a garnish. Lemon juice can be added for taste. This sauce was served over boiled potatoes or plain sliced meat.

Bilini with Cheese and Caviar

For Bilini; 1/3 cup buckwheat flour
2/3 cup all purpose flour
½ tsp. baking powder
¾ tsp. salt
¾ cup milk
1 large egg
1 stick butter

For cheese filling:
24 oz. cream cheese
2 eggs
3 T. sugar

Combine flours, baking powder and salt and mix. In another bowl whisk together the milk, egg and a tablespoon of the butter and then turn into flour mixture. Heat a bit of the butter in a hot skillet, and drip batter into the skillet, as for pancakes. Cook until bubbles form, about 2 minutes and flip until brown. They are now ready to fill with the cheese filling, which is placed along the centerline and heated for half a minute; then rolled, and served with a dollop of sour cream, and caviar. Smoked salmon can also be substituted as a filling. Ummmmm.

Berta's Colombian Sopa de Nidos de Golondrinias (Swallow's Nest Soup)

3c. Water
3 grated cloves of garlic
3 fine stems of green onions
Cilantro
Salt
Add all to the water; Add eggs to the water
Be sure not to break the yolks. Boil for 2-3 minutes. Crumble one cup
of French bread and 3 cups milk. Boil and then add Cilantro leaves
as garnish.

Plum Kuchen: (Baba made this for all of our birthdays)

1 c.butter
1½ c. sugar
4 eggs
2 c.flour
8 plums
1 t. cinnamon

Place butter in a bowl; rinse in hot water.
Add ½ cup sugar and 2 eggs at a time..
Stir briskly
Add the other two eggs (beat)
Add flour and spread in a deep plate
Bake 375 degrees for 30 minutes; serve with home-made whip cream.

Apple Kuchen- This was prepared for any and every occasion possible.

2 eggs
2 Tbs orange juice
1 c. sugar
½ c. butter
¾ tsp vanilla

Combine the above ingredients. Mix well. Add 1.5 cups flour, 1.5 tsp. baking powder. Mix well. Place batter in a greased, 10-inch kuchen dish.
Place 2 cups sliced apples on top of batter. Mix 3 tbs sugar and 1 tbs cinnamon and sprinkle on apples. Bake at 350 for 1 hour.

Mr. Happe's Meatloaf

A mix of ground pork, venison, and turkey to total 2 lb.
I package of Lipton onion soup mix
Sprigs of fresh rosemary, mint tarragon, basil cut fine (dry ok)
1 egg
¾ cup cornmeal or wheat bread toasted and broken into crumbs
Fresh onion chopped
1/3 cup celery chopped
1 Tbsp. worsteschire sauce

Mix all ingredients into a loaf shape
Bake in cooking dish at 350 degrees for one and a half hour

Russian Herring and Beet Salad (Maria's Christmas Specialty)

1 jar pickled herring in wine sauce
1 16 oz can of slice beets
¾ can of chopped dill pickles
1 can of small whole potatoes chopped
1 cup sour cream
Dash salt and pepper
1 Tbsp. capers
½ onion chopped

Cut the herring and place in a medium bowl. Add the beets, pickles, potatoes and sour cream, salt and pepper to taste. Garnish with capers.
Refrigerate one hour before serving. Serve in fine crystal bowl if possible!

Pickled Cucumber Salad

2 large cucumbers
1 tsp. salt,
¾ cup white vinegar.
1 tsp. sugar
¼ tsp. white pepper
2 T. fresh dill

Scrub the waxy skin off of the cucumbers and dry them. Score with a fork and slice very thin. Place in a colander and sprinkle with salt. Press with dry paper towel or clean kitchen cloth to drain after they have sat for about an hour or so. In a salad bowl, add vinegar, sugar, salt, and pepper and pour this over the cucumber and stir in fresh dill. Chill and Serve.

Plant Sorrell Soup

2 T. oil
1 qt.vegetable stock
8 cup Sorrell leaves
1 cup. Sour cream
Salt

Heat oil, celery, and bell peppers for 10 minutes. Add stock, sorrel, and parsley…. boil. Reduce heat and simmer for about 30 minutes Puree in blender with cream as sour cream, salt, pepper. Sugar can be added for taste.

Cherry or Plum Wine

Pounds of ripe plums or cherries
3 pounds sugar
1 small yeast cake or a package of active dry yeast
A handful of grapes or blackberries

Cook plums or cherries into a large steel cooking pot and cover with water. Set over medium heat and boil gently, then cook for 30-
 40 minutes. Remove from the stove and cool. Press the cooled fruit into a jelly bag and into a large glass container. Measure a gallon of juice and add 3 pounds of sugar. Stir and add yeast. Tie the jar with a clean white cloth and leave for 3 weeks. After 3 weeks pore into sterilized bottles and discard sediment. Cork and age for 6 months more.

Kulich/ Easter Coffee cake with Nuts and Raisins

3-5 cups of flour
½ cup raisins
¼ cup rum
2 cups confectioners sugar
1-cup warm milk
½ tsp. sugar
1 tsp. vanilla extract
10 egg yolks
½ tsp. saffron
½ cup silvered almonds

Pour ½ cup of the warm milk into a bowl and sprinkle with yeast and ½ tsp. sugar. Let the mixture stand for 3 minutes, then stir to dissolve the yeast. Set bowl in warm place, as an oven until it doubles in volume. Soak the raisins (light raisins are best). Pre heat the oven to 400 degrees and sift the sugar and 3 ½ cup flour over the missing bowl. Add the yeast mixture and ½ cup milk until the batter is formed. Beat in the vanilla and egg yolks.
Knead it by hand so it becomes smooth and elastic.

Then remove the raisins from the rum and spread them on paper towels to drain. Dissolve the saffron in the rum and pour over the dough. Knead the dough until all the liquid is gone. Place the ball on a lightly floured area, and knead for 10 more minutes adding flour as needed. Place it in a lightly buttered bowl and dust with flour, covering it with a kitchen towel, then placing it in a warm place until the dough doubles in volume…Toast the almonds for 5 minutes or so…After it has risen, place the dough in a greased and floured coffee can (2-4 may be used depending on their size) and fill them to no more than 1/3 full. Allow the dough to rise again for another half hour…Then Bake for 1-1 ½ hours at 300 degrees until it is golden.

Baba Ghanoush (No, it was not named after Maria)

1 eggplant
2 cloves garlic, minced.
1 ½ tablespoon olive oil
Salt and pepper to taste

Preheat the oven to 400 degrees. Lightly grease a baking sheet.
Poke holes in the eggplant with a fork and then place it on a baking
sheet. Roast it for 35 minutes until soft. Turn once or twice. When it
is soft, remove from oven and place in cold water. Skin should peel
of easier now. Place eggplant into blender and puree, with added garlic and salt and pepper. Place mixture in a bowl and stir in olive oil.
Refrigerate a few hours before serving.

Spinach and Nettle Soup

Handful of young Nettles
1 small onion
1-2 cloves garlic
1 pkg. fresh Spinach
1 can chicken broth
3 oz cream cheese

Melt one Tbsp. of olive oil and one of butter. Add onion and garlic
and sauté in pan until tender. Wilt nettles and spinach. Add broth
and softened cream cheese. Bring to a boil. Puree in smaller batches
and serve warm.

Grape and Curry Chicken Salad (Maria's luncheon favorite)

4 skinless boneless chicken breasts cooked and diced
1 diced stalk of celery
4 chopped green onions
1 diced apple
1/3 cup golden raisins
1/3 cup grapes cut in half
½ chopped toasted pecans
Black pepper to taste
1 tsp. curry powder,
¾ cup light mayo

In a large bowl, combine chicken, celery, onion, apple, raisins, grapes, pecans and mayonnaise. Mix all together and then add spices and mix once more.

Pashka; Russian Easter Dessert: (This goes with the Kulich bread)

This was an essential dish in a Russian Orthodox home and one can use the mold made of wood or plastic, Maria would just mold it into a dome shape by hand.

2 pounds dry curd or farmer's cheese
5 large egg yolks
2-¾ cups confectioners' sugar
1-cup heavy cream
½ cups coarsely chopped almonds
½ cup golden raisins
1 cup candied citron
2 tsp vanilla
½ pound, 2 sticks unsalted butter

Pass the farmers cheese through a sieve and set aside. Mix egg yolk and sugar in a double boiler and then add the cream. Heat until bubbles form around the edge of the pan. Stir constantly. Remove from heat and add cheese, almonds, raisins, citron and vanilla, mixing well. Add butter and continue stirring until it cools. Line it with damp cheese-cloth and pour the mix inside. Place a small plate on top to weight it down. Place a bowl underneath to catch the run off and refrigerate for 24 hours. Remove from mold and decorate with jellybeans, almonds, candies of sort, citron or flowers and leaves. Slice and serve!

Braised Red Cabbage

1 T. olive oil
1 large chopped onion
2 large peeled and sliced carrots
1 large head red cabbage, cored and sliced to ¼ in. thick
1 large green apple, cored and sliced.
3 large clove garlic
1 bay leaf crushed
¼ tsp. ground cloves
1 ½ c. dry red wine
¼ c. red wine vinegar

2 T. light brown sugar
1 c. peeled chestnuts

In a large pot heat the olive oil. Add onion, carrots and sauté. Add cabbage, apple, and mix together. Add salt, garlic, bay leaf, cloves, wine, vinegar, sugar, and bring all to a boil. Cover and cook one hour.

Violeta's Salsa Mexicana

3 ripe tomatoes
1/3 c. chopped onion
1–3 chiles, serranos or jalepenos
½ c. chopped cilantro
2 Tsp. salt

Combine tomatoes, onion, chiles, cilantro and salt in a sauce dish. Stir

Maria's War Story

By Anna Sypula -
Friend and Former Journalist

As Poland fell under the influence of the Soviet Red Army, two tall, unusually dressed women quietly crossed the German border into British controlled territory, bringing with them an icon from the private chapel of Alexandra, the last Empress of Russia.

It was hot that May in 1947, but the two women wore coats with several dresses underneath. They were accompanied by a man in his early 20s and a hunchbacked woman, who helped them to escape.

Before they started their long and dangerous journey which took them through Polish woods and the underground tunnels of East Germany, one of the women, Lili Dehn (Maria's mother), sewed into the lining of her clothing her greatest treasure – letters written by the Empress just months before the whole imperial family was murdered in Ekaterinburg.

These letters had a special meaning to Dehn. They were written to her and were part of her memories of the days she spent in Tsarskoe Selo with her dear friend, Alexandra. They reminded her of her own arrest in Tsarskoe Selo and of the heart-breaking moment when Alexandra, together with her husband, Nicholas II, an several of their five children gathered around her to say good-by for the last time.

In the spring of 1947 when Dehn and her 23-year-old daughter Mary, climbed out of an underground tunnel that brought them into a field controlled by British soldiers, they also had photographs of the Imperial family and a precious medallion hidden in their clothes.

The photographs were given to Dehn by the czar's children, who upon hearing the news of her arrest ran into their rooms and returned quickly and thrust them unto her hands. It was then that the Empress placed a little medallion on Dehn's neck and said the words Dehn never forgot –"Lili, by suffering, we are purified for Heaven. This goodbye matters little. We shall meet in another world."

Today these items are the most treasured possessions of a Bethesda resident, Dehn's daughter, Maria Happe She helped her mother smuggle them out of Poland and after Dehn died in 1964 she brought some of the to the Washington D.C. area.

The Icon of Christ that once was a centerpiece of the Empress's own chapel, now shares space with the photographs on the Tsar's family in the Happe's split-level colonial house. The back of the icon still bears an inscription written by Alexandra.

Alexandra's personal chapel has been described in several well-known books. For example, biographer Robert K. Massie offers a picture of the chapel in his bestselling "Nicholas and Alexandra".

"To the right of the bed a door led to a small chapel used by the Empress for her private prayer," writes Massie. "Dimly lit by hanging lamps, the room contained only an icon on one wall and a table holding a Bible."

The icon was later given to Dehn by Alexandra as a symbol of their friendship, according to Dehn's book "The Real Tsarista."

Today, this icon as well as photographs and letters have become relics for Dehn and her family. They are placed behind glass doors of the china cabinet in a corner of the living room. Although most of the photographs have faded, Alexandra's signatures and inscriptions still can be seen quite well. Amazingly, the icon seems untouched by the series of the turbulent events it witnessed – first civil war in Revolutionary Russia, then World War II in Poland, and finally three escapes to the West.

There were many situations in which Dehn was close to losing all her treasures. Maria witness one such drama in 1944, when she and her mother tried to cross the eastern front and get to the West.

"We were stopped by the Red Army," recalls Happe. "They took all the stuff we had and threw it out on the snow. I remember looking at the snow and there were all these letters of the Empress, her pictures and little souvenirs my mother received from her. The soldiers never knew what it was. They were looking for money and other valuable things. When they walked off, my mother quietly picked everything up."

Tough at the time, the soldiers sent the two women back to Poland, they had at least one reason not to despair – part of their valuable possessions had survived their unsuccessful escape.

In 1918, when Lili Dehn was ready to leave Russia, she had a number of objects that came from Alexandra. She received them on various occasions: Christmas, birthdays, and just as a sign of their friendship. Alexandra, who was the godmother of Dehn's son Alexander, always sent him numerous gifts.

As Dehn's son described it in his unpublished memoirs, Christmas Eve was always a special time, because "towards the evening two special couriers sent by the Empress from the palace would arrive with a huge carton about six feet long, and four feet high, containing presents for me. I particularly remember a large mechanical music box, a balalaika, toy soldiers, and lots of clothing..., which had belonged to the throne Grand Duke Alexis, who was my playmate, and who was four years older than I."

When Alexandra's godson, whom she affectionately called "Titi" was baptized, she presented him with a beautiful golden cross encrusted with diamonds and an icon.

Alexandra always cared about her Godson. Even in the midst of Siberia, where the whole Imperial family was kept under house arrest, she wrote letters to her "little Titi."

When life in the Bolshevik Russia became too dangerous, those letters and the cross left Russia with Dehn.

In 1918, she carefully packed the precious items she had and joined an exodus of Russian aristocrats to the West.

Together with her then 10-year-old son, ailing mother, and a maid, Dehn waited for hours for a train on a dirty and crowded platform. When the train finally arrived, they were tossed into a wild crowd. Elbowing their way to the train, they didn't notice that in the chaos of boarding they had left something behind. It wasn't until later that they noticed that one of their suitcases was missing.

"They looked out of the window and there I was standing on the platform," recounts Happe. "They has the most valuable things in it, many of which came from the Empress. The train was already moving and there was no way that they could get off and pick it up."

The train was gaining speed. It was heading to Odessa, a port city in the Southern Ukraine. As any journey in those difficult days, their trip was fraught with dangers.

"The train was about to pass a station called Znamenka, when we were warned that the place was occupied by bands of separatist Ukrainian troops led by the anarchist Machno, and that we would have to break through the station at full speed with the hope that the line ahead was clear," Dehn's son writes in his memoirs. "We flew through the station with all machine guns and rifles firing, and we were lying on the floor behid sacks of oats. The enemy likewise opened fire. Several bullets entered our boxcar, but Providence was with us, and there were no casualties. We managed to get through."

The trip, which under normal circumstances would have taken 10 hours, lasted 11 days. When they reached Odessa it was already packed with thousands of refugees. There were rumors that Bolsheviks would soon arrive. Dehn made every possible effort to obtain passage on a ship, which was about to leave for Constantinople, in Turkey.

After bribing a few officials with some of her jewelry, she got the passage.

As the ship was leaving the port, passengers saw motorized columns of Bolshevik troops moving from the East into the city.

As soon as Dehn got to Constantinople, she tried to find out if her husband was alive. In 1916, he had been an officer on the imperial yacht, the Standart, when Nicholas II ordered him to go to Japan and bring the battleship "Variag" to England for convoy services there. Later the same year Dehn's husband became the commander.

After considerable time and trouble she got permission to go to England. When the cargo ship Dehn boarded was approaching the port of destination, a small motor boat hurried in their direction. A tall blond man in a grey civilian suit climbed up the ladder. The captain of the ship greeted him and then came up to Dehn and her son.

"'Mrs. Dehn, here's your husband Captain Dehn,' the captain of the cargo ship said, turning to my mother," Dehn's son recounts in his memoirs. "My mother must have nearly fainted from joy, as neither of us had recognized in the clean shaven civilian, my father, whom we had last seen in a Russian Naval Uniform, with a large blond moustache."

It was in England that the Dehns decided to sell the diamond cross given to their son by Alexandra. "It was well sold," remembers Happe. "My mother wanted my brother top go to a private school." He did, before fate brought the Dehns to Poland, where they lived until their escape in 1947, then to Venezuela and finally to the United States.

After their successful escape in 1947, when they arrived in Venezuela, the Dehns had little money. To start off life in their new homeland, they needed basic things, such as an icebox and a car. They bought these things with the money Happe's mother got from selling a diamond brooch created by the famed Russian court jeweler, Peter Faberge. According to Happe, it was first pawned in a shop and later sold to the wife of the President of Venezuela.

At the same time, several old French miniatures were sold as well. However, Dehn never sold the icon or Alexandra's letters. "She treasured them," says Happe.

As the letters from Alexandra faded and became weather-beaten, Dehn decided to deposit them at Yale University, which she did in the early 1960s.

Out of those letters, Dehn sold only one. She wanted to help her long-time friend, Anna Vyrubova, with whom she had spent many happy days with Alexandra in Tsaskoe Selo. She sold the letter to Marjorie Merriwether Post. Authorities recognize that Vyrubova and Dehn, were Alexandra's most intimate friends. They often were intermediaries between Alexandra and Gregory Rasputin, a ragged "moujik," who is said to have used tremendous hypnotic powers to stop severe hemorrhages that the hemophilia-stricken tsarevich suffered from. In 1917, while with Alexandra and her family, the two women were arrested together by Alexander Kerensky, then the head of the provisional government.

In the early 1960's, Vyrubova lived in inland with very little money and was in poor health. "I remember we mailed her about $500 after the letter was sold," Happe recalls.

Shortly afterwards, the little medallion that Alexandra gave to Dehn during their last meeting, was gone, too. When Dehn died in 1964, Happe put it into her mother's coffin. "I knew she wanted to have it with her," Happe says.

Among the treasures that still are in the possession of Dehn's daughter is a little photograph of Nicholas and Alexandra, which was taken before they were engaged.

"It's upstairs. I will show it to you," says Happe, turning to her guest. "It has never been published."

Struggle

A man found a cocoon of an emperor moth. He took it home, so that he could watch the moth come out of the cocoon. One day, a small opening appeared, and he sat still, watching for several hours, as the moth struggled to force its body through the little hole. Then, it seemed to stop making any progress. It appeared, as if, it had gotten as far as it could and it could go no farther. It seemed to be stuck. Then, the man in his kindness, decided to help the moth.

So, he took a pair of scissors, and snipped off the remaining bit of the cocoon. The moth then emerged easily. But, it had a swollen body and small, shriveled wings. The man continued to watch the moth, because he expected, at any moment, the wings would enlarge and expand to be able to support the body, which would contract in time. Neither happened! In fact, the little moth spent the rest of its life, crawling around with a swollen body and shriveled wings. It never was able to fly.

What the man, in his kindness and haste, did not understand was, the restricting cocoon and the struggle, required for the moth to get through the tiny opening, were God's way of forcing fluid from the body of the moth, into its wings, so it would be ready for flight, once it achieved its freedom from the cocoon. Freedom and flight would only come after the struggle. By depriving the moth of a struggle, the man deprived the moth of health.

Sometimes, struggles are exactly what we need in our life. If God allowed us to go through our life without any obstacles, He would cripple us.We would not be as strong, as what we could have been.

Author Unknown

"Alles gut, Endes gut..."

(Kurt's saying)

CPSIA information can be obtained at www.ICGtesting.com
Printed in the USA
BVOW11s1626310714

361021BV00009B/52/P